The Back Pain Bible

Other books by Anthony J. Cichoke, M.A., D.C.:

Bromelain (A Keats Good Health Guide)

The Complete Book of Enzyme Therapy

Enzymes and Enzyme Therapy: How to Jump Start Your Way to Lifelong Good Health

Enzymes: Nature's Energizer (A Keats Good Health Guide)

Introduction to Chiropractic Health: Achieving the Body Balance That Can Defend Health and Protect Against Chronic and Acute Diseases, 3d edition

The Back Pain Bible

ANTHONY J. CICHOKE, M.A., D.C.

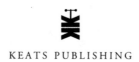

KEATS PUBLISHING

LOS ANGELES

NTC/Contemporary Publishing Group

The Back Pain Bible is intended solely for educational and informational purposes and not as medical advice. Please consult a medical or health professional if you have any questions about your health.

Library of Congress Cataloging-in-Publication Data
Cichoke, Anthony J.
The back pain bible / Anthony J. Cichoke.
p.   cm.
Includes bibliographical information and index.
ISBN 0-87983-903-1 (pbk.)
1. Backache—alternative treatment.   I. Title.
RC771.B217C49   1999   99-31339
                                                      CIP

Published by Keats Publishing
A division of NTC/Contemporary Publishing Group, Inc.
4255 West Touhy Avenue, Lincolnwood (Chicago), Illinois
60646-1975 U.S.A.
Printed and bound in the United States of America

International Standard Book Number: 0-87983-903-1

10 9 8 7 6 5 4 3 2

Contents

Preface

This book can help you eliminate back pain. It is a bible of techniques developed and successfully used to rehabilitate my neuromuscularly handicapped son, David, and thousands of other back pain sufferers.

What is a bible? It is a lifetime road map, a philosophy of life, to be read and reread, to be used and internalized, to be shared with family and friends.

Those of you who have heard me speak or have read any of my other books are aware of the tremendous role that David and my other children have played in my personal and professional life. Although I was interested in health during my early years, my focus intensified and crystallized by the fight to rehabilitate David after he suffered a serious brain and back injury in a fall at three years of age. Diagnosed with acute cerebellar ataxia, he had severe neuromuscular problems with poor coordination, and he suffered much back pain. He walked like a child with cerebral palsy. The doctors gave little hope; he could need a wheelchair or be bedridden all his life. Eventually, he was released from the hospital, not because he was cured, but because they had no rehabilitation program for him. There really wasn't anything that could be done—or so the doctors said. David's future looked very dark.

Only through a power far greater than mine and a program developed with the assistance of world-renowned doctors, psychologists, nutritionists, exercise physiologists, and people of the spirit were my wife and I able to rehabilitate David. Eventually, I realized that yes, David had suffered a physical injury, but the injury was causing emotional and nutritional stress as well. Only by balancing all three factors—the physical, nutritional, and emotional—were we able to return him to health. Over the years, David fought back and overcame his physical disability. We watched David become a national honor student and a world-class athlete. I have since used the techniques that worked so well with David to help thousands of my patients free themselves from the shackles of back pain and live healthy, happy, productive, and pain-free lives.

From my thirty years as a practicing chiropractor, from my work with David, and from my extensive research, I have learned that wellness and harmony come from within the body. Fortunately, more and more physicians in the United States are beginning to accept this concept and recognize its value. The Chinese, of course, have understood this philosophy for thousands of years—it is an integral part of Traditional Chinese Medicine (TCM). Practitioners of TCM, as well as many holistic health care practitioners in this country, know that disharmony and imbalance can cause disease and dysfunction. In many cases, this dysfunction leads to back pain—a condition that plagues most of us at some time in our lives.

My purpose in writing this book is to help you win your battle over back pain. This book will teach you to identify your enemy (the cause of your back pain) and will show you how to defend yourself against the emotional, physical, and nutritional stressors that assault you every day, throwing your body out of harmony and balance and leading to pain, depression, and illness. By blending the best of TCM and Western natural medicine, I will show you how to control and defeat your demons and, in the process, how to discover your inner self, return your body to harmony, and conquer your back pain—all without drugs or surgery.

Acknowledgments

The author wishes to thank the following researchers and physicians for their cooperation, advice, assistance, and information in writing this book: Raul Ahumada, Edward Alstat, Motoyuki Amano, Takahiko Amano, Vladimir Badmaev, W. Bartsch, Wayne Battenfield, D. J. A. Cole, Tony Collier, Michael Culbert, F. W. Dittmar, James Duke, Charles Fox, Naritada Fujiki, G. Gallacchi, G. Gebert, Wilhelm Glenk, Yoshihide Hagiwara, Clare M. Hasler, John Heinerman, A. Hoffer, Rudolph Inderst, Hans Jager, Peter Karnezos, Leslie Kenton, Shigeki Kimura, Franz Klaschka, Gert Klein, Michael W. Kleine, Stephen E. Langer, Benjamin Lau, Joe Lehmann, Robert I. Lin, D. A. Lopez, T. Pearse Lyons, Muhammed Majeed, E. J. Menzel, Mark Messina, John Mills, Earl Mindell, Daniel B. Mowrey, Michael Murray, Tracey Mynott, Sven Neu, Christine Neuhoffer, Richard A. Passwater, Otto Pecher, Barbara Pfannenschmidt, Joseph Pizzorno, Joan Priestley, H. D. Rahn, Karl Ransberger, Vic Rathi, Corey Resnick, Robert Rosen, W. Scheef, Ed Schuler, Art Sears, J. Seifert, Lendon Smith, G. Stauder, C. Steffen, Peter Streichan, Koichi Suzuki, Mitsuru Takiura, Steven Taussig, G. P. Tilz, Ron Tominaga, Klaus Uffelmann, Wolf Vogler, W. Von Schaik, Morton Walker, R. Michael Williams, Heinrich Wrba, Janet Zand, and finally Ms. Katie Cichoke and William Cichoke.

A huge thanks goes to the libraries of America and especially to Portland, Oregon's West Slope Library for their hard work, support, and neverending cooperation.

Special thanks to my secretary, Mrs. Karen Hood, for all of her assistance in the preparation of this book, including doing research, typing, and editing; to proofreader Beata Szewezyk; and to Peter Hoffman, Nancy Kolodny, and Claudia McCowan of Lowell House/Keats Publishing for their special work as editors.

Finally, my eternal thanks to my wife, Margie, for her neverending support and for enduring the mountains of paper and manuscripts in our house for these past two years.

How to Use This Book

This book is divided into three parts. Part 1 explains the incidence of back pain, who is most likely to suffer from back pain, and when you should see a doctor. Part 1 also presents a brief explanation of the mechanisms of the spine, the way pain occurs, and the role the rest of the body plays in keeping the spine and related nerves, muscles, tendons, and ligaments healthy and happy. Because this book is a marriage of Eastern and Western philosophies, part 1 also explains Traditional Chinese Medicine (TCM) and holistic medicine. Part 2 describes the emotional, physical, and nutritional factors that can cause back pain. Part 3 explains the Five-Step Jump-Start Plus Program, a treatment program that merges the principles of my Five-Step Jump-Start Program (first described in my book *Enzymes and Enzyme Therapy: How to Jump Start Your Way to Lifelong Good Health*, published by Keats in 1994) with those of TCM and other philosophies of the Eastern world. This part focuses on the various steps you can take to cure your back pain and prevent future flare-ups through stress relief, detoxification, diet, supplements, exercises, and physical techniques. It also gives you specifics on how to increase your body's innate healing potential.

As you read this book, keep in mind that everyone is different and that no treatment plan will be effective without a firm commitment from you. Conquering your back pain requires making the appropriate emotional, physical, and nutritional changes in your life. Without that commitment, permanent success cannot be achieved.

This program takes willpower and desire, but it's fun! Remember, however, that consistency is the secret to success.

Once you get on the program, you won't give it up. It will burn fat and give you increased energy and better muscle tone. It will enhance your life and give you spirit, confidence, and increased personal power.

Regardless of your size, shape, or age, *The Back Pain Bible* works! With this program, you will experience and enjoy a deeper appreciation of the universe around you and the wholeness within you.

Part One

Back Pain: What's Going On?

Back Pain: Just How Big of a Problem Is It?

Does it feel as though the entire Green Bay Packer football team danced all over your back? Are you bent to one side like a broken weather vane after a tornado? Is your back as stiff as a piece of leather in a Minnesota blizzard? If so, join the group.

Did you know that 80 percent of us will experience back pain at some time in our lives[1]—and that the remaining 20 percent will know someone with back pain? This means that every single one of us will be directly or indirectly affected by back pain. Back pain is impartial and does not discriminate. It crosses all socioeconomic, racial, age, and religious lines.

Back pain is a serious problem experienced by people all over the world and it appears to begin early in life. One study indicated that by the time girls were eighteen years old and boys were twenty, more than half of them had experienced low back pain at least once in their young lives![2]

In the United States, national statistics indicate that 15 to 20 percent of the total population will suffer from low back pain this year alone.[3] A survey of working-age people found that they have it even worse. Half of this group experiences back problems every year.[4-6]

Back symptoms are the second leading reason patients give for seeing their physicians.[7] According to a recent article in *Spine*, there were almost fifteen million office visits for low back pain alone in 1990.[8] Males forty-five to sixty-four years of age had the highest number of visits to a physician, while men fifteen to sixty-four years of age saw a physician more frequently than did women of the same age.[7] The most frequent diagnosis was strains and sprains, followed by rheumatism and arthritis, intervertebral disk problems, and diseases of the urinary tract (the symptoms of which often include back pain). Women were less likely than men to have back injuries.[7] See Table 1.1 for a look at the course of back pain throughout life.

Back pain is expensive. A recent article estimated that several billion dollars are spent every year on the treatment of low back pain in the United States.[9] In fact, the cost of treating low back pain is six times higher than the cost for AIDS-related illnesses, which tend to be very expensive in their own right.[9] In addition, back problems frequently cause time lost from work.

But back problems can affect more than just your pocketbook. They can decrease your ability to enjoy or perform normal activities and can cause profound disability. In fact, for those under the age of forty-five, back problems are the most frequent cause of disability.[10] Almost 1 percent of the U.S. population is chronically disabled from back problems at any given time.[3] That doesn't sound too bad until you realize that in 1994 the U.S. population was 260 million.[11] This means that 2,600,000 people were chronically disabled, at least temporarily, because of back pain. And the problem is growing. According to the U.S. Bureau of Census, the projected population of chronically disabled people could jump to a tragic 2,723,300 people by July 1, 1999.

If you're reading this book, it's probably because you have back pain. You already know how it has affected your life, how daily activities that used to be so simple—like taking out the garbage or bending over to pick up something off the floor—are now either painfully impossible or at least very uncomfortable to do. You also know the monetary cost of your back condition.

Table 1.1

BACK PAIN THROUGH LIFE

WHEN BACK PAIN OCCURS	WHAT'S HAPPENING
Pregnancy	Increasing weight downward and forward pulls and stresses the lower back.
At birth *(mother)*	The mother's body (and back) experience violent muscle contractions.
At birth *(child)*	Birth can be a violent and traumatic experience to the baby's body.
Early childhood	When born, the child's entire spine is C-shaped backward. As the child develops and begins raising her head, the neck becomes C-shaped forward. Eventually, the lower back becomes C-shaped forward.
Adolescence	Changes in life can cause subluxations and developmental problems.
Athletics *(trauma and stress)*	Football, basketball, baseball, and other sports can all cause trauma and place stress on the back.

(Continued)

Table 1.1 *(Continued)*

WHEN BACK PAIN OCCURS	WHAT'S HAPPENING
Injuries and accidents *(at work, home, or recreation)*	Physical injuries can directly affect the spine, causing pain and leading to metabolic changes.
Aging	Joint stiffness and weakening of the bones (osteoporosis) can occur with increasing age.
Chronic disorders	Osteoarthritis and rheumatoid arthritis can adversely affect joints throughout the body, including those of the spine.

WHO IS MOST AT RISK?

People who are overweight and those who do heavy lifting or frequent bending are likely to experience low back injuries. Individuals whose occupations demand repeated lifting, particularly in a forward-bent or twisted position, are at especially high risk. One study found that people whose jobs required repeated lifting of objects weighing more than about 25 pounds over twenty-five times a day experienced a greater than threefold risk of rupturing a lumbar intervertebral disk than those people whose jobs did not involve such activity. Also, the risk was increased with fewer repetitions if the person also twisted while lifting. Furthermore, lifting heavy objects in a twisted position without bending the knees resulted in an especially high risk of prolapsed lumbar disk.[12] Warehouse workers, delivery people, and grocery clerks (among others) frequently do this type of lifting. You may be lifting objects in excess of 25 pounds on a daily basis without even thinking about it. If you twist sideways leaning into your car to extract your 25-pound squirming toddler, you increase your risk for back problems.

How about sports? Do they increase your risk of back pain? It seems obvious that those who participate in sports such as hockey, football, gymnastics, golf, bowling, and snowboarding have an increased risk for low back injury. Over the years, I have treated many athletes for their sports-related injuries.

Certain occupations seem to increase your risk for back problems. Many of my patients were long-haul truckers and others who sat for extended periods behind the wheel or were exposed to vibration (including vibrating industrial machinery). Those who suffer from developmental or congenital spinal conditions (such as osteochondrosis, spondylolisthesis, and spinal stenosis) also have an increased incidence of back pain, as do those suffering from osteoporosis.

The causative factors mentioned here are all physical factors that increase an individual's susceptibility to back pain. However, there are other factors, such as nutritional deficiencies and emotional stress, that can disturb your body's balance and set you up for back problems. The bad news is that if you have ever suffered from back pain before (regardless of the cause), the odds are great that you will suffer again.

RAPID REVIEW

- As many as 80 percent of us will experience back pain, and the remaining 20 percent will know someone with back pain.
- Back pain appears to begin early in life.
- Repeated lifting of objects as light as 25 pounds can cause a low back disk to rupture.
- Overweight individuals are more prone to back problems, as are those whose jobs involve heavy or repeated lifting, bending, or twisting.

To beat back pain, you need to understand the role that nerves, muscles, tendons, ligaments, and bones play in back health. That's the subject of chapter 2.

Two

Understanding Your Back Pain

P ain is a protective mechanism. It is your body's way of alerting you that something is wrong. Fortunately, most cases of back pain are not permanent or serious, and the pain goes away on its own in a few days. Unfortunately, we cannot always take a break when our back has had too much. Life must go on, work must continue, even if our back hurts. But remember—back pain is a warning sign. Its purpose is to force you to react and remove yourself from the cause of the pain. If you ignore the pain signals and fail to remove the cause of the pain, the problem can worsen and become chronic, causing serious consequences throughout your entire body.

In the body, pain—whether sharp, stabbing, pricking, boring, burning, aching, or throbbing—is detected and transmitted to the brain by nerves. Nerves are cordlike bands of tissue, primarily composed of fibers. They are the telephone wires of the body responsible for transmitting pain signals to the brain. The brain is like a huge building of telephone operators and switches. The brain and spinal cord (the body's major highway for nerve transmission) compose what is called the *central nervous system*. Thirty-one pairs of nerves come from the spinal cord and pass to the body through openings called *foramina* (singular, *foramen*) between the vertebrae. This includes eight pairs of cervical nerves, twelve pairs of thoracic nerves, five pairs of lumbar nerves, five pairs of sacral nerves, and one pair of coccygeal nerves. These nerves, in turn, branch out and spread throughout the body. This "outer portion" of the nerve network makes up the *peripheral nervous system*, which is quite extensive. In fact, the total length of peripheral nerves in the human body is about 93,000 miles.[1] Pain can occur anywhere along these nerve pathways.

Your brain, the nerve control center, is constantly receiving signals from nerves throughout the body. Most of the time, these signals are ignored. It is estimated that 99 percent of the sensory information received by the brain is discarded as unimportant. For example, unless you take the time and effort to think about your clothes, and unless they're restrictively tight, most of the time you're unaware of the feeling of the clothes on your body. Similarly, when sitting, you are unaware of the pressure of your body on the chair.

However, the brain pays attention when it is in the body's best interest to do so. For instance, if you were to burn your hand on the stove, pain receptors would transmit a signal to the brain. Acting much like a complex computer, the brain would sort through the technical data, decide not to discard this information, and return a message to the injured area: "Move your hand off the hot stove."

VERTEBRAL SPINE

In addition to supporting your body from the head to the lower back, your bony spinal column plays a very important role in protecting the spinal cord from injury. The back is composed of thirty-one bones, called *vertebrae*, twenty-four of which are movable. There are four major sections of the spine:

■ *The cervical region* is composed of seven vertebrae in the neck that doctors like to number C-1 through C-7. The main characteristic of the seven cervical vertebrae is their exceptional flexibility. These vertebrae support the head, and their mobility allows the head to have a wide range of motion in turning to the left and right and looking up and down—almost like a swivel.

- *The thoracic spine* (midback or dorsal region) is composed of twelve vertebrae numbered T-1 through T-12. Vertebrae in this area attach to the ribs with special ligaments. This area of the spine is relatively immobile because of the rib attachments.

- *The lumbar region* (lower back) is composed of five vertebrae called L-1 through L-5. The lumbar spine carries the majority of the weight of the upper body. These vertebrae are heavier and broader than the ones above in order to support the large body mass, as well as the very large muscles attached to these vertebrae. This area also is implicated in many neurological conditions of the low back and of the legs, because many nerves leave the spine in this area. The lumbar curve is the hardest working part of your spine because it carries most of your weight.

- *The sacral and coccygeal region* is composed of the sacrum and the coccyx (tailbone). The *sacrum* is an upside-down, triangular structure that constitutes the base of the spine. The sacrum is broad and is attached to the lumbar vertebrae. The sides of this wedge-shaped structure attach to the pelvis. It begins in the developing embryo of the mother's womb as five separate vertebrae. As time passes, they fuse and a single bone (the sacrum) is formed. Below the sacrum is a collection of a few small bones, called the *coccyx* (pronounced "cox-ix"). This is hypothesized to be the remnant of the tail we humans possessed earlier in the course of our evolution.

Although the upper three vertebral curves are flexible enough to bend and twist, the vertebrae of the sacral and coccygeal region are fused in the adult (but are flexible in earlier years). These vertebrae must be properly aligned for a healthy, pain-free back. This is because these natural curves support you when you move and act to evenly distribute your weight throughout the spine, thus reducing your chance of injuring your back.

INTERVERTEBRAL DISKS

The vertebrae in each of the three movable sections of the spine (the neck, midback, and low back) are cushioned and separated by disks. These intervertebral disks are like soft cushions, or pads, that separate the bony vertebrae and serve as shock absorbers. The spongy center of the disk is called the *nucleus pulposus*. It is surrounded by a tougher outer fibrous ring called the *anulus fibrosus*. The disk is a lot like a jelly doughnut—a soft center surrounded by a firm outer ring. Back flexibility, as well as the ability to move and bend, is accomplished through the movement of fluid within the nucleus. This allows your vertebrae to rock back and forth on your disks.

Fibrous cushions, the intervertebral disks act to pad and maintain the space between the twenty-four movable vertebrae. These twenty-three cushionlike pillows make flexibility of the spine possible (and are critical for normal movement) but act in much the same way as shock absorbers in a car or the springs in a mattress. Your disks are constantly under stress—expanding and compressing, turning, twisting, and torquing.

VERTEBRAL LIGAMENTS

Ligaments are bands of fibrous, thick, and very tough strands of tissue. In the body, they serve to attach one bone to another and also strengthen and support joints like hinges on a door. Many ligaments in the spine connect and hold the vertebrae, the pelvis, and the sacrum together. Ligaments are flexible but not very elastic; they can be stretched only so far before they rupture (an overstretched ligament is called a *sprain*). Think of ligaments as a series of rubber bands holding a group of children's blocks together. They'll stretch only so far before they give out. Once stretched beyond their limit, they can never return to their original size or shape.

VERTEBRAL MUSCLES

Muscles move bones. They are responsible for every move you make. Through a cycle of tension (contraction) and relaxation, muscles produce movement in a specific area of the body. Contraction is initiated by nerve impulses, which also control the intensity, rapidity, and relaxation of your muscles. Muscles can go through this tension/relaxation cycle for an indefinite period. Spasms and pain develop, however, if a muscle is under sustained tension without an alternating relaxation phase. This tension can develop from poor posture, certain repetitive movements, emotional stress, nutritional deficiencies, or injury. Sustained, continual tension can keep the muscles from relaxing and can set you up for back pain.

There are approximately 640 muscles in the musculoskeletal system.[1] In fact, more than 40 percent of the body's weight is composed of the musculoskeletal system.[2] Any one of these muscles can develop spasms, be injured, or become overly fatigued. A *strain* occurs when a muscle is overstretched.

Maintaining the strength and flexibility of several different muscle groups is of particular importance to a healthy back. This is because, in addition to their role in movement, muscles provide support for the entire body and help to keep the spine erect. Weakness in any muscle group can lead to back pain. To illustrate this concept, imagine that you are erecting a four-sided tent, using ropes at each corner for support. To hold the tent vertically erect, each rope has to exert a pull equal to that of the other three. If one rope is slack or weakened, the tent will not remain vertical, no matter how strong the other three ropes are. The extent to which the tent sags or even collapses will depend on the slackness of the weak rope.

Your spine acts in much the same way. If one muscle group is weak because of lack of exercise, poor nutrition, disease, paralysis, injury, poor posture, or poor body mechanics, body balance will be disturbed and your structure will weaken. This, in turn, will affect associated ligaments, nerves, tendons, and other muscle groups. Damage to the spine and organs can result.

The exercises presented later in this book are targeted to improve the flexibility and strength of muscles and are a key part of any rehabilitation program.

TENDONS

Tendons are similar in structure to ligaments, but they have a different function. Unlike ligaments, which attach one bone to another, tendons attach muscles to bones. However, like ligaments, tendons can be overstretched and torn, causing inflammation of the tendon (a condition called *tendonitis*) and pain.

THE VICIOUS CYCLE OF BACK PAIN

Back pain occurs when nerve endings near the spine receive abnormal stimulation. These signals are transmitted from whatever area is affected—be it vertebrae, muscles, tendons, or ligaments—to the brain, where they are interpreted as pain. As a result of the perceived back pain, a reflex action occurs in the back. Muscles go into spasm in an attempt to protect the back and to keep the damaged area immobile. If prolonged, the muscle spasms can result in a vicious cycle of even further stiffness and pain as our once healthy and balanced four-sided tent collapses.

We all react differently to pain. Some people can tolerate very little, while others can tolerate a great deal. The problem arises when we ignore the pain signals our back is sending.

If you held a lit match until the flame reached your fingertips, you would feel pain and immediately drop the match. The pain is a warning sign to move your fingers from the heat source. But with back pain, we can't easily remove ourselves from the source of the pain because (1) we often don't know why our back hurts and therefore don't know what to change and (2) our back goes everywhere we go. But by not removing the cause of the pain, we set ourselves up for a vicious cycle of muscle spasms that lead to pain, which then increases the muscle spasms that cause more pain.

WHEN TO SEE YOUR DOCTOR

With back pain, there are times when you must see a physician for examination, consultation, and possible treatment. Seek treatment immediately if any of the following occurs:

- If your pain is due to a traumatic injury, such as a car accident
- If your back hurts during or after a fever or illness
- If you suffer from tingling, numbness, or weakness in the legs, especially below the knees and into the feet
- If your pain is constant, nagging, and neverending, even when you change position (lying, standing, or sitting)
- If your pain is accompanied by bladder and bowel problems
- If you can't walk on your toes without the whole foot dropping to the floor

RAPID REVIEW

- Think of the spine as a shock absorber, a coiled spring supporting the weight of the body. It can flex, extend, bend, rotate, and withstand the shock of your daily activities, all the while protecting the essential spinal column from injury.
- The spine is composed of thirty-one vertebrae.
- Intervertebral disks act as cushions for the vertebrae.
- All messages from the brain pass through the spinal cord, which runs through the spine to vertebral nerves and out to the organs and cells of the body.
- Ligaments help hold the spinal vertebrae together.
- Muscles, whose fibers are like many rubber bands expanding and contracting, allow your vertebrae to flex, extend, bend laterally, and twist. These muscles act like the restraining cords of a four-sided tent, keeping the structure balanced. Emotional, physical, and nutritional stress can cause spinal muscles to weaken, leading to imbalance and pain.

Western medicine sees back pain as very simple—it is caused by some kind of problem affecting the vertebrae, disks, ligaments, muscles, or tendons. These problems are most often addressed by drugs or surgery. But holistic physicians, and much of the rest of the world, do not view health, disease, or pain as many do in the West. Traditional Chinese Medicine (TCM), for instance, views back pain as being caused by a disruption in the flow of *chi* (vital energy), leading to disharmony and imbalance. This is the subject of our next chapter.

Part Two

How Your Lifestyle Is Causing Your Back Pain

Three

Traditional Chinese and Holistic Medicine

The previous chapter introduced terms like *vertebrae, muscles, tendons, nerves,* and *disks.* This was necessary to give you landmarks for your road map back to health. Torn tendons, stretched ligaments, pulled muscles, and inflamed nerves can all pull your body out of balance and lead to back pain.

A physician in the United States might say that your back pain was caused by a slipped disk or strained back muscles. To relax the muscles and relieve the back pain, such a physician might prescribe pain killers or muscle relaxants. In some cases, surgery might even be suggested. That's because Western medicine often fails to see the whole, the totality of a human, and instead sees the body as fragmented pieces, like a broken mirror to be glued back together through surgery and drugs.

Traditional Chinese Medicine (TCM) is a holistic medicine, viewing an individual as a complete entity. That is, no single part of the body can be understood as a separate component but must be viewed in relation to the whole. Symptoms are seen as part of the totality of one's entire bodily pattern and not related to one specific causal condition. Eastern medicine regards the symptoms in one part of the body as a local manifestation of the burden placed by a disorder on energy throughout the body. That is, the symptoms are a reflection of disorder in the whole body.

TCM is keenly aware of balance and what happens to the body when balance is disturbed. Understanding the Eastern concept of balance is essential to fight illness and return your body to health. According to TCM, body imbalance is the cause of illness and back pain.

Bodily wellness is experienced when one is "in harmony"— that is, in mental, physical, and nutritional balance. Distressing symptoms are only a segment of complete bodily imbalance that mirror, or reflect, other aspects of life and behavior.

TAO

Tao is a Chinese word meaning "way" or "path." More literally, Tao is a path one walks by following one's head as opposed to one's feet. Tao is a philosophy of life in which one is guided by the mind, not the body. Although it is Chinese in origin, Tao has universal applications and was the cornerstone for TCM. Taoism is an ancient Chinese philosophy that teaches people the value of their health and emphasizes harmony with nature.

CHI

All organs in our body require energy. The TCM term for energy is *chi* (pronounced "chee"). This term is sometimes written *qi* or *chee*. In Eastern medicine, anything that interferes with the body's energy flow disrupts the process of healing.

Chi flows through the body through certain energy pathways or channels called *meridians*, which are somewhat like nerves. The body has twelve paired meridians (one on each side of the body). These energy pathways flow to vital organs of the body. Interference of energy flow through the meridians can cause imbalance and result in illness, such as weakened tendons, muscles, bones, or nerves, as well as osteoarthritis or rheumatoid arthritis.

Meridians

Meridians (the pathways through which chi flows) are divided into yin and yang meridians. Yin and yang are alternating forces that flow through all nature. Yin is the negative force, or pole, while yang is the positive force, or pole. These polarities are repeated constantly in nature: moon and sun, softness and firmness, sweet and sour, earth and heaven, woman and man, a magnetic positive and magnetic negative, quiet and motion. According to Chinese medicine, yin and yang are two faces of the same coin—not separate entities.

Examples of these opposites are seen everywhere in your body. For instance, when muscles such as the biceps contract, the opposite muscles, your triceps, should relax. In a healthy body, when you walk, one leg steps forward while the other stays back. Your arms have a similar movement. The left arm moves forward while the right arm moves backward.

Chinese philosophy sees a harmony and order within the body and throughout the universe. This harmony is achieved by maintaining a delicate balance between the opposing forces of yin and yang. If this balance is broken, chaos will occur. In the human body, this can result in pain and illness.

The back is our river of life. To survive, we need a strong back. For a river to survive, it needs a constant and steady supply of water. Adapting to our environment as water adapts to its environment can help us beat back pain.

Lao Tze, a Chinese writer and philosopher who lived almost twenty-five hundred years ago, discussed water and its ability to adapt in his book *Tao The Ching*. His concepts seem very appropriate in contemplating the imagery of water and our own ability to adapt to our environment. Lao Tze lived during one of China's most turbulent periods, known as the Warring States period. Water was one of Lao Tze's favorite images. Although water is all around us, according to Lao Tze it goes mainly unnoticed. It benefits all living things without being given credit for its accomplishments. Although it gives life to us all, water seems content to continually yield, to be flexible, to be soft, yet unrelentingly powerful. Please contemplate the following:

Nothing under heaven is more yielding than water;
But when it attacks things hard and resistant,
There is not one of them that can prevail.
That the yielding conquers the resistant
And the soft conquers the hard
Is a fact known by all men,
But utilized by none.[1]

This concept of water, softness, and flexibility is very important for us to internalize in the control and elimination of back pain. Our body, our mind, and our spirit must learn to yield and be flexible to let our "river of life" flourish.

Softness is a second concept of Lao Tze. The following passage is exquisite to contemplate. Note its implications for aging, stress, and life in general:

Man is weak and soft when he is born
He becomes hard and stiff, in death.
In life, thousands of plants, trees, and creatures are soft and supple.
Truly, to be hard and stiff is the way of death.
The way of life is to be supple and soft.
Therefore, the weapon that is too hard will be broken.
And the tree with the hardest wood will be cut down first.
Truly, the hard and strong are cast down
While the soft and weak rise to the top.[1]

This passage is a favorite for practitioners of China's "soft-style" martial arts. It trumpets the virtues of bending with the wind, of nonresistance, and of not being rigid.

There are many parallels that can be drawn from these passages in regard to back pain. With overwork, an injury to the back, disease, stress, or aging, our back becomes more rigid and less flexible, and the result is increased and more frequent back pain. By taking on the attributes of water and softness, we can better "give" with each stressful situation and be more flexible in body, mind, and spirit. Also, the way we approach all tasks in life should be armed with this golden "soft" and "fluid" rule of life. Follow this principle as you continue to use this book.

It is interesting that just as Lao Tze lived during a chaotic chapter in his country's history, so are we living in a chaotic period in our history. We need to be flexible if we are to survive. We must not be rigid. Therefore, Lao Tze's writings and philosophy speak to our own survival of body, mind, and spirit. In a way, Lao Tze gave the world a method of maintaining hope and surviving.

As you can see, the philosophies of TCM and Taoism are very different from those of Western medicine. However, they are similar in that their primary goal is to improve your health. Fortunately, more and more Western physicians are learning how important a healthy emotional state, proper nutrition, and physical conditioning are to improving back pain.

In the next chapter, we will discuss the emotional, physical, and nutritional factors in your life that disturb your body's flow of energy (chi) and can cause and perpetuate back pain. Once you recognize and understand the reason for your pain, you'll be better able to fight the pain, cure the underlying problem, and return to health.

In the following chapters, the concepts of Taoism and TCM will be interwoven with those of natural Western medicine. An emphasis on harmony and balance between opposites as well as balanced mental, nutritional, and physical health will form the key to all healing concepts and a practical foundation for building roadways leading to longevity.

RAPID REVIEW

- TCM treats the whole body and in doing so balances the body's yin and yang in returning you to health.
- Tao is the path, the philosophy of one's harmony with nature.
- All organs in the body require energy (chi) to function.
- Meridians are pathways through which chi flows.
- Tao teaches us to be like water and adapt to our environment.

Four

Physical, Emotional, and Nutritional Imbalances

requently, back pain comes on suddenly as a result of a car accident or work injury, lifting a heavy object, or some other type of physical stress. In addition, the body is subjected to emotional turmoil every day. We're all familiar with the emotional upset that a high-powered job, a troublesome teenager, rush hour traffic, or any of a million other things can produce. Emotional stress hits us from every angle, upsetting our body's delicate balance and causing perpetuating back pain.

Nutritional stress and imbalance can also cause back pain. If you eat the average American diet, you have reduced levels of key micronutrients such as vitamins, minerals, and enzymes. Your body was not designed to run efficiently on frosting-filled cupcakes and highly carbonated drinks loaded with refined sugar and caffeine. In fact, anything short of an optimal diet will leave your body unbalanced and more vulnerable to back pain.

Unfortunately, back pain often has no identifiable cause. Like a thief in the night, it can sneak up gradually, slowly developing into a constant, dull ache or an all-encompassing pain so severe that it brings your life to a standstill. When back pain has no obvious origin, it may be caused by an overlapping of emotional, physical, and nutritional imbalances (see Figure 4.1). Your body is no longer in harmony. Your flow of chi has been disturbed, resulting in pain and illness.

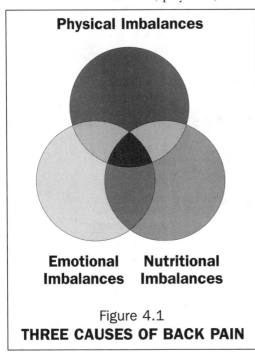

Physical Imbalances

Emotional Imbalances   **Nutritional Imbalances**

Figure 4.1
THREE CAUSES OF BACK PAIN

Many people think that the word *stress* refers only to nervous strain. However, stress is actually the way your body reacts to change of any kind. According to Hans Selye, M.D., considered the father of stress research, stress is the nonspecific response of the body to any demand. Whether this stress originates from external or internal sources— whether it is from emotional strain, nutritional deficiency, or physical injury—it is still stress, and it causes profound changes in the human body. The first step in permanently controlling back pain is to identify what's causing stress on your body, resulting in pain.

In 1956, Hans Selye published *The Stress of Life*,[1] in which he explains the general adaptation syndrome (GAS), or the stress syndrome. Selye claims that rather than affecting a specific part of the body, stress affects many parts of the body in a general sense. Actually, Selye developed the holistic theory without calling it such. According to Selye, the stress response affects the blood vessels, brain, connective tissue, glands (including the adrenal and thyroid), liver, nerves, and white blood cells. He also points out that we can combat pain and disease by strengthening our body's ability to fight stress.

Selye discovered that the body's reaction to stress consists of three stages. The first step is the alarm reaction. In this step, among other physical reactions, the adrenal glands are stimulated and enlarge, while the thymus and lymph nodes shrink. The body then enters the second stage, the stage of resistance. In this stage, the body tries to fight off the effects of stress. This includes attempting to cope with the wear and tear caused by the continual bombardment of life's pressures (whether physical, emotional, or nutritional). Inflammation is an excellent example of the body's efforts to resist a stressor (whether it be pathogenic or physical, such as muscle strain or ligamentous sprain). But if the source of stress continues, the body is beaten down and eventually enters the third stage, the exhaustion stage.

The human body has a very complicated mechanism of self-regulating checks and balances. Our body's innate capacity strives to maintain harmony and balance in keeping with the concepts of yin and yang. This machinery is incredibly efficient in helping the body to adjust to practically anything that can happen to us each day and throughout life. Unfortunately, this is not a perfect world, and our body's machinery is not always working at an optimal level.

Now that we've discussed how imbalances disturbing your body's harmony can cause health problems, let's look at the physical aspects of stress and how they affect your back and joint pain.

PHYSICAL IMBALANCES AND HOW THEY CAUSE BACK PAIN

Back pain often results from physical problems. Injuries, poor posture, disk protrusions, muscular problems such as fibromyalgia or strains, degenerative conditions (including arthritis), and poor muscle tone are only a few of the physical problems that can result in back pain. It can also be caused by interrelated factors because the muscles, ligaments, disks, and bones of the back are supplied by numerous interrelated nerve endings. Fatigue, anxiety, and stress can perpetuate back pain, and nutritional deficiencies can compound the problem.

Injuries

Injuries can result in several painful and serious back conditions, including a vertebral fracture or a ruptured disk. However, strains and sprains are probably the most frequent injuries resulting in back pain and are common conditions in the majority of back pain cases. Either or both can cause muscle spasms in the back, leading to inflammation and pain.

A *sprain* occurs when ligaments are torn, overstretched, or otherwise injured, while a *strain* occurs when these same events affect a muscle. A whiplash is a common condition that can involve both strains of the muscles and sprains of the ligaments. Most whiplash injuries occur in automobile accidents.

Although automobile accidents cause their fair share of back problems, many of the injuries we sustain are caused by our own foolish mistakes. And even the most fit individual can suffer from a back injury. Glen is a good example. Fifty years old and in top physical condition, Glen is a world-famous cross-country coach who has trained Olympians. His high school cross-country team has consistently won national honors. Glen first injured his back while attempting to pick up a heavy box. Not only did the resulting back pain interfere with his daily five-mile run and other physical exercise, it caused a total change in his lifestyle. Someone else had to take out the garbage, mow the lawn, move the furniture, and lift the groceries. This created a great deal of frustration for Glen. And it all could have been avoided if he had never attempted to pick up the box!

Just like Glen, many of us lift heavy objects or use poor body mechanics when lifting. We reach out too far from the waist when lifting and pick up heavy objects that we probably shouldn't be lifting anyway. Fortunately, Glen was in excellent physical condition and improved rapidly using my Five-Step Jump-Start Program.

Unlike Glen, many Americans are out-of-shape couch potatoes. For this group, improper lifting techniques are particularly dangerous because weak, flaccid muscles no longer support the body's frame. The sudden overwhelming stress of trying to lift a heavy object can cause tearing or stretching of the back muscle fibers and possibly even the ligaments. The capillaries (small blood vessels) and soft tissue cells in the area may rupture or tear. It is even possible to rupture a disk.

Heavy lifting triggers a number of physical and physiological changes that can accelerate damage to the disks. Remember, the disks' job is to cushion the bones of the spine. Damage to the disks can eventually cause back and joint pain and disability. Lifting causes compression of the disks, as shown in a recent study conducted by Jeffrey Lotz and associates at the University of California at San Francisco.[2] In their research, they found that the disks are actually destroyed when continually compressed. The greater the pressure, the larger the number of cells killed. With widespread cell death, the surviving cells' ability to repair and maintain the disks is eventually limited. This results in fluid loss inside the disks, and the disks become dehydrated. As a result, the disks are less able to withstand pressure and bulge outward. Disk dehydration triggers other changes, such as a release of chemicals that seem to irritate surrounding nerves. The pain associated with disk degeneration may be caused by the pressure that bulging disks exert on nearby nerves, coupled with this chemical release.

Ruptured Disks Severe injuries can lead to ruptured disks (also called protruded, herniated, or "slipped" disks). When disks bulge, tear, or rupture, some of the "jelly" can ooze through the side of the disk, decreasing the disk's ability to cushion the vertebrae and absorb shock, thus leading to some of the most common back difficulties. A disk problem can irritate or even pinch one of the nerves exiting from the spinal cord, often resulting in pain shooting down the leg, a condition called *sciatica*. This, in turn, can cause the rest of your spine to weaken, leading to pain, stiffness, and other symptoms.

Although injuries can cause this type of problem, so can degenerative changes. As we age, our disks tend to wear down and crack—just like a car tire. As the disks dry out, the spaces between them decrease in size. This causes the vertebrae to come in closer contact with each other, resulting in a decrease in the size of the opening (the *foramen*) through which the nerves pass. This can create friction and place pressure on the vertebral nerves, causing tremendous pain. The intervertebral foramen can also be narrowed by the growth of bony spurs (or bony outgrowths) that cause pain as the adjacent nerves are irritated.

Warning: If you suspect a disk problem, see a physician immediately. The longer you wait, the more serious could be the consequences. Luckily, surgery is not always necessary. Often this condition can be successfully treated with conservative methods, such as those found in this book.

Whiplash is another common injury affecting the spine and is a good example of what can happen when a ligament is injured. A whiplash is a cervical sprain that occurs when a sudden motion causes the head to whip one way and then the other, stretching and tearing the ligaments and muscles in the neck. A whiplash is usually caused by a car accident and can cause headache; neck, arm, and shoulder pain; weakness; numbness or tingling; dizziness; and visual disturbances such as double vision. In some cases, these and other symptoms might not appear for several hours or even days. This is because it takes time for fluid from the small blood vessels to seep into the surrounding tissue and cause the inflammatory process.

Whiplash injuries can cause tremendous trauma to the neck, including strains of the neck and shoulder muscles; sprains or tears of associated ligaments; subluxation, dislocation, or fracture of the vertebrae; disk herniation; and nerve and spinal cord injury. Left undetected and untreated, whiplash can result in permanent pathological and degenerative changes to the neck and other areas involved. If you suffer from a whiplash injury, it is critical that you immediately seek professional care.

Other Injuries That Can Cause Back Pain In addition to sprains, strains, and ruptured disks, fractures of the vertebrae can also cause significant back pain. Osteoporosis (meaning "porous bones") is a frequent cause of fractures in the elderly. This condition is marked by a loss of bone mass that causes deterioration of the spinal vertebrae or the weight-bearing joints such as the hips. Bones gradually thin and weaken, a process that leaves them highly susceptible to fractures. In fact, osteoporosis is usually diagnosed only after a person fractures a hip or one or more of the vertebrae collapse (this is called a *compression fracture*). Found predominantly in those forty-five years of age and older, this condition affects some 15 to 20 million Americans and each year causes an estimated 1.3 million fractures of the vertebrae, forearms, hips, and other bones.[3] Women are affected two to six times more frequently than are men.

Injuries can also cause a spondylolisthesis—a forward movement of the vertebral body (in relation to the vertebra below) and a separation in the vertebral part called the *pars interarticularis*. The term *spondylolisthesis* comes from the Greek word meaning "slipping vertebrae." When one vertebra slips forward, several vertebrae above it also seem to slip forward. The separation can be caused by an injury or may be present since birth and aggravated by an injury. You can control a spondylolisthesis, but it will never go away.

Sports and Back Pain Sports participation is a two-edged sword. On the positive side, sports can get you in shape and help keep you there, strengthening muscles important to back health. Sports can also teach you discipline and give you a sense of achievement and self-worth. The down side is that injuries and back and joint pain can become your constant companions. An example of this two-edged sword is the joint flexibility that often improves when you exercise. We know that flexibility is important to spinal and joint health, but moving joints beyond their normal range of motion (hyperextension) can undermine stability and strength.

Most of us have probably seen the commercial featuring a snow skier taking a particularly hard fall down a snowy slope while the announcer comments on his "agony of defeat." True, many sports are known for the trauma they inflict on participants. Broken bones, sprains, strains, and contusions are all part of the "game" and can all cause back pain. But a number of sports can lead to back spasms because of the unnatural posture a participant must assume in order to play the sport or because of the repetitive movement required in the sport. Golf is a good example.

I used to see a lot of golfers limp into my office. They frequently had low back pain because the twisting forces necessary to produce a swing powerful enough to drive a ball down the fairway place tremendous stress on the low back. The pain can worsen as the club hits the ball and the golfer "follows through" with his or her swing. At this point, golfers tend to hyperextend their backs, creating an inverted C. The cure? Try a more upright swing with not as much sideways bending.

A number of sports can cause back pain. Just consider the following list:

- Soccer, as well as football, basketball, rugby, and baseball, can cause nagging chronic back pain or acute traumatic injuries to the back. With the rough and tumble movements (running, turning, dodging, jumping, twisting), backaches can be unwanted companions.
- Although it seems obvious that a volleyball player would suffer stress and injury to the upper back, shoulders, elbows, and wrists, the rest of the body can also be affected. This is because the movement of body weight can transfer stress, sending shock waves down the length of the body and resulting in damage to the midback, lower back, knees, and ankles.
- Rowing often requires pulling on a single oar. However, this unilateral activity requires forward bending of the back, then a backward movement of the torso. This places a great deal of pressure on the neck and shoulders, as well as increased pressure on each subsequent intervertebral disk down the length of the spine to the tailbone.
- Figure skating not only puts stress on the ankles, knees, and shoulders, but puts stress on the back as well. The twisting and rapid turning and leaping all take their toll. For example, the lutz is a jump that is approached while skating backward. The skater pulls the upper body to the right, plants the right toe pick, and then swings the body forcefully to the left as he or she jumps into the air. To land, the skater must "check" the body, placing the arms strategically to stop the rotation. The contortion

necessary to complete this jump places incredible stress on the low back.

- In swimming, the two strokes that probably cause the greatest back pain are the butterfly and the breaststroke. The butterfly involves forcefully driving both arms forward over the head and then pulling them behind the body while undulating the low back. These movements cause constant stress to the back. Swimmers who practice the breaststroke tend to overdevelop their chest muscles. This overdevelopment can pull the shoulders forward, giving the swimmer a kyphosis, or "hunchback." In addition, the violent twisting and turning of flip turns can also be a source of back injury and pain for swimmers.

- Running is another source of pain to the back. Running puts repeated stress on the load-bearing joints of the ankles, knees, and back (especially the low back). Tight, cool muscles and improper running shoes can be a definite cause of joint and back injury. For this reason, stretching and flexibility warm-up exercises are critical before running, while cooldown exercises are essential following running. Nike, Adidas, Reebok, New Balance, and other companies have made a science of running biomechanics. For shoes and other equipment, check with a reputable store.

Remember, an ounce of prevention is worth a pound of cure. Sports are great, but they can be a two-edged sword. Following the stretching exercises in chapter 8 before and after any sports activity can help you avoid injury.

Posture and Balance

As the son of a chiropractor, I was fortunate to learn the importance of good posture early in life. Faulty body posture can cause one set of muscles to be overworked while another set is underworked, causing it to weaken or atrophy from lack of use and leading to muscular imbalance. Ligaments can be similarly affected, which can limit joint mobility. This can place pressure on the nerves near the joint, resulting in pain. Remember, any imbalance in the body can cause poor health and pain.

Poor posture can also place stress on the disks, causing them to wear out prematurely. If the central portion of the disk dries up, the disk can lose its ability to cushion the spine. This creates a wide variety of spinal problems that can be avoided by correcting unhealthy postural habits.

Poor posture can result in abnormal deposits being laid down within the joint structure, which can then affect circulation to the joint. This chain of events can lead to a genuine case of arthritis. In this way, faulty body posture can cause a specific symptom complex or disease to develop.

Unfortunately, proper posture is not always easy to maintain. Unlike other mammals, humans don't have the structural advantage of the four-legged stance that spreads an animal's weight evenly over its body. In the human, gravity increases the pressure on the vertebrae from the head downward, with the stress being the greatest in the lower back. Since the low back supports the upper body, it is constantly under strain and vulnerable to injury. Poor posture increases this vulnerability because it places tension and pressure on the spine and can create a muscular imbalance.

Poor posture can be aggravated or even caused by foot problems, including flat feet, pronated feet, sore feet, or any problem that affects the feet and toes, such as corns or bunions, causing you to stand or walk differently. Knock-knees and bowlegs can also affect your posture because they cause the hips to rotate. This places extra pressure on the low back, tensing the muscles and leading to spasms and pain.

Poor posture disturbs the body's center of balance so that its self-righting mechanism must work overtime to keep you upright. To understand this concept and the importance it plays in back health, try a little experiment. Stand in front of a chair and place your right foot up on the seat of the chair. Notice how your low back adjusts to the right to keep you standing instead of leaning over? Your trunk and head also angle slightly to keep you straight.

This self-righting mechanism requires that your muscles be flexible and balanced to allow the spine, neck, and head to adjust and keep you upright. Without proper muscle movement, the body cannot align itself. Your nerves must also be healthy to transmit messages to the muscles, and your bones must be strong to support the spine. This allows the spinal nerves, arteries, and veins to pass vital messages and nutrients to and from the body's organs and cells.

The body's self-righting mechanism can actually create back problems if it is forced to compensate for a physical abnormality or weakness. This can cause an exaggerated curvature in various parts of the body as you attempt to self-right, leading to muscle spasms and pain.

The feet, pelvis, torso, cervical spine, and head are all involved in proper balance. For example, a foot pronation can lead to exaggerated curves, including an anterior (forward) tipping of the pelvis, a hunched back (thoracic kyphosis), and a forward movement of the neck and head. Foot pronation is a condition in which the foot rolls inward onto the arch, resulting in a flat foot that is often wider and longer than a similar foot with a proper arch. The body's weight falls on the arch, weakening the foot's supporting qualities. This also causes the knees to rotate inward. Hip rotation becomes abnormal and the Achilles tendons bow in. Each step causes a twisting stress to be placed on the pelvis. Ultimately, this can overstretch the supportive ligaments of the hip and pelvis. In an attempt to stay upright, the individual's pelvis moves forward, which then causes the shoulders to round and the neck and head to suspend outward. In fact, there is a tenfold increase in muscular effort on the part of the cervical spine for every inch of forward movement of the head and neck.[4] The body makes these adjustive movements in an attempt to stay upright, but this mechanical action can ultimately lead to muscle spasms and chronic pain.

An anatomically short leg can also affect the spine because it places strain on the pelvis and low back, leading to scoliosis, degenerative changes, or chronic pain. This condition can be easily remedied with heel lifts or other orthotics.

Even high heels can cause this kind of exaggerated, compensatory curvature. High heels force the body's weight onto the toes, shorten the hamstrings, and cause the low back to sway (a posture called a *lordosis* or *swayback*) as the wearer tries to stay upright. The shoulders hunch and the neck and head move forward to compensate. No wonder women suffer from back pain when they wear high heels! This same type of postural correction occurs when a woman is pregnant: The weight of the baby pulls on the low back, forcing the mother to make self-righting corrections to stay upright.

Even eyeglasses can cause postural problems and back pain. Anyone who now wears bifocals or trifocals probably remembers the struggle to adjust to these lenses. Individuals wearing multifocal lenses actually hold their heads more forward than those who don't wear such lenses.[5] Habitually placing the head out in front of the body's center of gravity can cause musculoskeletal and neurovascular dysfunction and resulting pain.

Scoliosis can be a severe postural problem. Scoliosis is an abnormal curvature of the spine—a condition commonly observed in children and teenagers (girls more than boys). Scoliosis can often be corrected by improving the individual's posture. Structural scoliosis can be congenital, but it is generally not considered genetic.

Regardless of the cause, scoliosis can put added stress on the body and cause back pain. Nerves that pass through the openings between the vertebrae and transmit messages to the body and to the brain may be irritated or even pinched. Disks, the shock absorbers of the spine that are located between the vertebrae, may wear down, rupture, or bulge. The muscles may become weak on one side of the body and overused or tight on the other; the base of the spine (called the *sacrum*) can be tilted and not level. If scoliosis persists into adult life, it can worsen and may affect adjacent organs in the body, such as the lungs and heart. All children should be screened periodically for scoliosis during their growth period. If you suspect scoliosis, see a physician.

Physical deformities such as scoliosis are often accompanied by poor body image and poor self-image. In many instances, the emotional pain can be more severe than the physical pain. Every mirror, every human eye, seems to accentuate and crystallize the problem. As previously mentioned, emotional stress can perpetuate a back problem.

CHECKING YOUR BODY'S BALANCE

First, look at yourself in a full-length mirror. Attach a string (the length of the mirror) to the top of the mirror near the middle. The string will act as a plumb line; gravity forces it to hang straight. Stand facing the mirror, directly in front of the string. From top to floor, the string should bisect the center of your body, dividing it into two even halves. It should run from the center of your head, through the center of your nose and mouth, down the middle of your neck, through your breastbone, through your navel, between your legs and ankles, and finally rest directly between your feet. If the string does not run straight down the centerline of your body, your body is not in balance.

Now, imagine you have a line drawn from ear to ear, eye to eye, shoulder to shoulder, and hip to hip. These imaginary lines should be level and run parallel to the floor. If they are at a slant, then you're not in balance.

Because the body attempts to balance itself in relation to the force of gravity, any deviation in posture is an indication of disharmony in the body and the result of the body's attempt to compensate. In recognizing any distortions or deviations in your posture, you are taking the first step to reversing this disharmony.

Gait Irregularities Poor posture and balance can cause gait irregularities that in turn can lead to more back pain. Gait refers to the manner or style in which we walk. Sometimes our gait is the cause, and at other times the effect, of a back problem. For instance, if you suffer from sciatic pain or hip pain, you may limp or shuffle your feet because each step causes pain. You may be bent to one side. Sciatica can also cause an individual to have an uncoordinated and unsteady walk, stepping down on the heel first and then onto the toes with a kind of double tap. When standing, the person's feet may be spread wide apart for balance.

On the other hand, an uneven gait might actually cause a back problem. Next time you are near a college, observe the uneven gait and bent posture of a student carrying a large, heavy backpack. This behavior can cause muscles to be pulled out of balance, leading to back pain.

Neurological Disorganization and Cross-Crawl The body's coordination is directed and controlled by the nervous system in a complicated and miraculous manner. When you walk, the nerve endings in your legs, feet, and lower body send nerve messages up to your brain and to the muscles of your upper back, shoulders, and neck to coordinate the activity of walking. But these nerve receptors can be impaired because of an acute, traumatic injury, from stretching or lifting in excess, or from many conditions that cause back pain. When this happens, the information may be garbled and confused, leading to gait problems.

In many ways, the gait problems caused by nerve, tendon, muscle, and ligament injury can mimic those caused by brain injury. Glenn Doman, founder and head of the world-famous Institute for the Achievement of Human Potential, in Wyndmoor, Pennsylvania, has done tremendous work with brain-injured children using a technique called *cross-crawl*. This technique involves lying face down and simulating the movements involved in crawling. His technique is instrumental in teaching brain-injured children how to walk.

I first used the cross-crawl technique with my son David, and I saw measurable improvement within a few months. He progressed from crawling to creeping and then to walking and finally running. Since then, I have found that the same cross-crawl techniques that worked so well with David are also helpful in improving the gait irregularities that often affect individuals with back pain—individuals without brain injuries but who suffer from nerve interference. Cross-crawl helps to improve the brain-body connection and therefore helps to improve coordination of the arms, legs, head, and neck.

In my opinion, each of us should use cross-crawl exercises on a regular basis, literally from womb to tomb (I will explain how in chapter 9). We all can have decreased brain and nerve transmission to some degree for varying reasons. A child, for example, may have delayed or abnormal creeping, crawling, and walking behavior relating to decreased brain function or nerve transmission. As adults, injury or pain can inhibit our ability to move our legs, to walk, and to move our arms in a synchronized fashion. This causes abnormal movement patterns to develop; muscles lose their ability to sense and react to abnormal situations and to work in mutual synergism with other muscles. An impaired or broken nerve circuit, which can be caused by a back injury, sprain, or strain, can also result in nerve interference. Messages just won't get through the motor pathways, or if they do, the messages may be faulty. Therefore, the normal synchronized movement will be impaired, resulting in irritation to the back and back pain.

This decreased function will continue until normal nerve pathways are restored, and this can be accomplished with the cross-crawl exercises in chapter 9.

Muscular Problems

Sometimes, physical sources of back pain develop gradually over a period of time, rather than suddenly, as from traumatic injury. Chronic muscle tension from repetitive motions or prolonged stress can cause muscle strain or muscle spasms—frequent reasons for back pain.

Myofascial pain syndrome (MPS, also called fibromyalgia, muscular rheumatism, or fibrositis) is a condition marked by muscle pain, tenderness, and stiffness. Any of the fibromuscular tissues can be affected, but those of the occiput (the bone at the base of the skull), neck, shoulders, thorax, lower back, and thighs are most common. MPS may cause chronic lower back stiffness and pain and may be associated with well-defined tender points, fatigue, muscle strain, stress, anxiety, or nonrestorative sleep, with or without inflammation. MPS can be caused or worsened by stress of any kind, including poor posture, poor sleep, emotional factors, nutritional deficiencies, injury, viruses and other infections, and exposure to cold or damp conditions.

Tight or shortened hamstring muscles can also cause back pain. The hamstring muscles run along the back of the thigh. If you exercise and don't cool down afterward, numerous muscles in the body, including the hamstrings, can tighten or go into spasm. In addition to being the effect, muscle imbalance can also be the cause of tight hamstrings. If the quadriceps (the muscles in the front of the thigh) are overdeveloped or overworked (as often occurs in runners), they can create a muscular imbalance and lead to tight hamstrings; they shorten and pull on the low back when they tighten.

Arthritis and Other Degenerative Conditions

As we age, our skin begins to wrinkle, our hair may turn gray (or fall out!), and we begin to develop many chronic disorders, including arthritis and rheumatism. The wear and tear of life decreases the body's ability to function—and the body begins to degenerate. The vertebrae become more porous as we age and can easily fracture. Over time, weight, pressure, and irritation can cause lipping (the development of bony overgrowths) and spurring of the vertebrae, which can place pressure on nearby nerves and arteries. In addition, the disks that cushion and separate the vertebrae can dry, harden, and crack, decreasing the size of the foramen through which the nerves pass. These and other degenerative effects can cause back pain.

Arthritis is probably the most common degenerative condition. There are actually two major types of arthritis: osteoarthritis and rheumatoid arthritis. Osteoarthritis is an inflammatory problem primarily affecting the weight-bearing joints, such as the spine, hips, sacroiliac, and knees, causing intense pain. At first the pain may increase with exercise, although exercise, and especially swimming, can actually improve the stiffness that may occur because of inactivity. The involved joints may swell or be warm to the touch. In this disease, the protective joint cartilage at the ends of bones gradually wears away, particularly in the spine and legs. Without the protective cartilage, the surface of the bones becomes exposed and the bones rub together. Bone spurs develop and can damage nerves and muscles. The end result is bone deformity, with pain and restricted movement.

Rheumatoid arthritis (RA) is a chronic inflammatory condition that specifically affects the synovial membranes of the joints but can also involve the entire body. The joints typically involved in this disease are the feet, hands, knees, ankles, wrists, and those of the spine. Characteristic symptoms include vague joint pain, joint stiffness, low-grade fever, fatigue, and general weakness. These symptoms can appear several weeks before the onset of swollen and painful joints. RA is an autoimmune disease—that is, the body's immune system is attacking the body itself. Although its onset may be abrupt, RA usually begins gradually. It can begin at any age, but the average age of onset is between twenty and forty. Approximately 1 to 3 percent of Americans are affected by RA, and females outnumber males by a margin of nearly three to one.

Inactivity and Lack of Physical Fitness

One of the primary reasons for back pain is simple inactivity and flabby muscles. As mentioned in chapter 2, strong, flexible muscles are of key importance in back health. Muscles provide support for the entire body and help to keep the spine erect. Weakness in any muscle group can lead to back pain. Many of the exercises in chapter 9 are designed to help strengthen the abdominal and back muscles and provide support for your back.

Infections

Sometimes back pain can be a symptom of some other problem in the body. Such is the case with a kidney infection, whose symptoms include severe back pain. There can also be tenderness along the vertebrae and between the ribs. Pain from kidney disease usually occurs in the side or back between the top of the hips and the last rib. The pain may even radiate up to the area of the stomach. Additional symptoms of kidney infection include nausea, vomiting, fever, and chills. Anyone with a kidney infection should be under the care of a physician.

INFLAMMATION

Pain? Swelling? Heat? Redness? Loss of function? These are the cardinal signs of inflammation. Inflammation accompanies many back and joint conditions, including sprains, strains, arthritis, fibromyalgia, disk problems, and other musculoskeletal problems. If you were to cut your finger and the wound began to hurt and then became red, hot, and swollen, you would clearly see the signs of inflammation. This same process can occur in the organs and tissues of your body, including the muscles, tendons, and ligaments near the spine. Inflammation of this type can cause a significant amount of pain and discomfort, regardless of its origin.

Viewed biochemically, inflammation proceeds in three gradual and partly overlapping phases. In the first phase, the body reacts to the injury. The capillaries initially dilate, causing them to be more permeable. This is why we often bruise when we're injured. Eventually, blood and other fluids accumulate in the injured area. This buildup keeps nutrients and oxygen from getting in and waste products from getting out, resulting in swelling of the tissues. This stage can last up to three days. In the second phase, which typically lasts from three days to six weeks, the body begins the reparative process. During this phase, the body continues to eliminate any abnormalities and attempts to restore normal function. It does this by first restoring the necessary microcirculation of the capillaries. Proper circulation improves the delivery of beneficial nutrients and oxygen to the injury site and also helps the body eliminate the highly toxic products resulting from trauma or infection. During the third, or regenerative, phase (which lasts from three weeks to twelve or more months), the body makes its final effort to correct and repair the damage by filling in the area with scar tissue.

The speed at which inflammation occurs and is resolved is regulated in the body by hormonelike chemicals called *prostaglandins*. Within the body there are both "good" and "bad" prostaglandins. The "bad" prostaglandins stimulate pain receptors, cause pain, and encourage inflammation, whereas the "good" prostaglandins inhibit inflammation and decrease pain transmission.

Physical trauma, emotional stress, or nutritional stress can upset the delicate balance between the two types of prostaglandins. When this occurs, the body produces large amounts of "bad" prostaglandins, overwhelming the "good" prostaglandins and preventing the body's defense mechanisms from acting properly. Only when the original balance is restored can healing take place.

Overweight

I remember one patient particularly well. Mary was a very large woman who came to my office suffering from severe low back pain. As part of her treatment program, I recommended a weight loss plan, because obese patients with back problems can be extremely difficult to treat. Excess weight is a threefold problem. First, excessive weight causes the spine to be less flexible, keeping the shock-absorbing curves of the spine from "giving" when they need to. Second, the increased weight can decrease the size of the foramina—the vertebral openings through which nerves and arteries pass—causing a pinched nerve or artery. Finally, and possibly most important, the potential for complete low back recovery in an obese patient is greatly decreased because the weight of the abdomen is continually pulling the stomach and lower back forward and downward. This results in a severe hyperlordosis (an increased forward curve) and misaligned vertebrae, which are frequent problems in the obese.

According to the National Institutes of Health, ninety-seven million American adults are overweight.[6] Besides being at increased risk of illness from type II diabetes; lipid disorders such as high cholesterol; circulatory disorders, including hypertension, stroke, and coronary heart disease; osteoarthritis; gallbladder disease; respiratory problems; certain cancers; and sleep apnea, these individuals, just like Mary, also often suffer from back pain.

Back pain has become the "disease of civilization." Our modern lifestyle is much more sedentary than that of our ancestors. Instead of working in the fields, most of us sit at our desks during the day and in the evening plop down in front of the television. We have become couch potatoes and have the excess pounds and back pain to prove it. Unlike our ancestors, we eat nutritionally dead fast foods. And with today's fast lifestyle, we are under constant and increasing stress. We're stressed, out of shape, and overweight. No wonder we have back pain!

EMOTIONAL IMBALANCES AND HOW THEY CAUSE BACK PAIN

When we are ill, our body is trying to get rid of excessive negative energy and destructive forces. One of the main problems could be psychological, or emotional, stress. Therefore, we must discover the nature of the obstruction—the negative force that is causing disharmony. Frequently, we have suppressed unpleasant memories. These memories can block our ability to attain harmony. Freeing ourselves of these emotional obstructions can be essential in returning us to health and releasing us from the clutches of back pain.

John is an excellent example of the effect that emotional turmoil has on the body. John, accompanied by his wife, came to my office complaining of neck and shoulder pain. The muscles in his neck and right shoulder were extremely tight and tense, so much so that his neck was pulled slightly to the right and his right shoulder was elevated. He was examined, treated, and his pain relieved. As he walked out into the parking lot in front of my office, he began arguing with his wife. Their loud voices caused me to glance out the window. As I watched them walk away, I could actually see John's right shoulder begin to elevate and his head tilt to the right. Emotional stress can cause physical problems. It can also increase your risk for cancer, hypertension, atherosclerosis, and stroke. The great news is that stress can be managed and need not be hazardous to your health.

Emotional stress can be the feeling of anxiety or stimulation you feel in a new, old, or challenging situation. It can energize you or depress you. How you emotionally perceive an event can affect your body's physical response to that event.

High-pressure work at the office or in school, ringing telephones, noise, traffic, and competition in every phase of our lives keep us in a high state of emotional stress. According to Dr. Archibald D. Hart in his book *Adrenaline and Stress*, stress sets off a chain of physical responses in the body.[7] It first causes the pituitary gland in the brain to release adrenocorticotrophic hormone (ACTH), which in turn stimulates the adrenal glands. At the same time, the brain sends nerve messages to the adrenal glands as well as other areas of the body. The adrenal glands then release a number of hormones, including cortisol, cortisone, adrenaline, and noradrenaline, that cause an increase in arterial pressure and blood flow to active muscles. At the same time, blood flow to organs, including the stomach and kidneys, decreases, while cellular metabolism throughout the entire body increases, as do blood glucose concentrations, mental activity, and muscle strength. The body triggers this increase in nervous and hormonal activity to allow us to perform far more strenuous physical activity than might otherwise be possible. This reaction is called the *fight-or-flight reaction*, and an important part of this stress response is increased muscle tension. Noradrenaline alerts the muscles to tense up and get prepared for quick action, which is why we have greater strength and can move faster in response to danger or a threat.

The fight-or-flight reaction worked well in our evolutionary past, when our ancestors had to decide in a split second whether to stand and fight the saber-toothed tiger or run away as fast as their legs would carry them. Unfortunately, in today's civilized world, we can't always run away or take a stand and duke it out. We effectively live lives of caged animals with minimal opportunities to respond to outside irritations. If you're an hour late for work and get pulled over for speeding, your options do not include running away or fighting with the traffic cop. Nor can you punch out your boss if he's giving you a bad time. Your body, however, has been programmed by thousands of years of evolution to respond to stress by providing the hormonal and nervous energy to run away or fight. So instead of doing either, you simmer. Blood flow increases to your brain, your heart beats faster, your blood pressure rises, your stomach secretes extra acid, your hands begin to sweat, and there is increased tension in your muscles. This muscle tension remains even if no action occurs. The body adopts an "on guard" posture—that is, shoulders up with arms slightly forward. Take a look in the mirror at your body language the next time you're angry or upset. This "on guard" posture lasts as long as a person feels threatened.

Because we do not have the same outlets through heavy exercise as our ancestors did, and because civilization does not approve of the natural response through fight or flight, our muscles store up the tension. This constant tension deprives the muscles of elasticity and shortens them. Muscles under sustained tension that are not allowed to relax will eventually develop pain and spasms. This increased tension can cause back pain, as well as headaches, a stiff neck, shoulder pain, teeth grinding, sore jaws (such as occurs in temporomandibular joint [TMJ] syndrome or pain), and generalized leg and arm pain. In this way, emotional stress can lead to actual physical problems, including back pain.

In addition, over time, we develop conditioned responses to specific events. If we are faced with the same type of problem over and over again, our body's defenses, as well as our emotional, physical, and metabolic reactions, may become stereotyped. For example, let's assume you have a particularly obnoxious math professor. Each time he calls you to the chalkboard to demonstrate a problem, he makes a fool of you. After a few episodes, your nervous system learns what will happen once you reach the chalkboard. So, in anticipation, your pulse speeds up, your palms sweat, and you feel sick to your stomach. This will happen even though—just this once—he's giving you an award for tremendous improvement. Your nervous system reacts automatically in a trained and conditioned manner, just as Pavlov's dogs did in his famous study on salivation. In any conditioned response, the body tends to react to a stressor in the same way, time after time, regardless of whether the response is appropriate to the situation.

Chronic, unrelenting muscle tension can also cause muscles to deteriorate, setting the stage for the first episode of back pain. Even the simplest act of picking up a pencil or a piece of paper may cause the first attack of back pain. This leaves the muscles stiff and weakened and predisposes the back for the next painful attack, which in turn will compound the symptoms. The vicious cycle has begun!

What Research Shows About Emotional Stress and Back Pain

Although researchers do not yet understand all the mechanisms involved in how stressful life events cause back pain, they do know that emotional stress is at the core. A recent study compared two groups of patients suffering from back pain. The first group had an organic basis for their pain, while the second group had pain of uncertain origin (idiopathic pain). Significantly more patients with idiopathic pain had at least one highly stressful event before experiencing pain. This group was greatly more exhausted and had significantly more difficulty in coping with the stressful events in their lives.[8] This shows just how much of an influence stress is in causing back pain.

Further, the makers of the drug Nuprin conducted a survey of pain in the United States and found a very strong relationship between pain and stress and between pain and hassles.[9,10] The greater the hassles and stress, the greater the severity, frequency, and incidence of all reported pains. Stress was mentioned voluntarily by study participants as a major cause of backaches, menstrual and stomach pains, and headaches (but not pain in the joints or muscles or dental pain).

To overcome emotional stress, you must first learn to identify it. In fact, attention to the body's signals is critical in controlling back pain. Unfortunately, stress may interfere with your attention to the body's pain signals, increasing the possibility that you may stand, move, or sit in ways that cause strain to the muscles. Further, stress can negatively affect any rehabilitation or prevention program because emotional stress can make you feel like giving up. In fact, when under stress, most people discontinue their exercise programs—an important part of any rehabilitation program. By doing so, any strenuous work they perform may cause them to further injure their already weakened body.

It is possible to combat emotional stress and remove any factors that may be causing or perpetuating your back pain. Chapter 7 will teach you how to regain your emotional balance.

NUTRITIONAL IMBALANCES AND HOW THEY CAUSE BACK PAIN

Nutritional imbalances can contribute to back pain, in part because diet plays an important role in conditioning your responses to stress. A poor diet can leave your body without the nutrients it needs to properly function. Inadequate nutrition sensitizes the body to anti-inflammatory corticoids and can lead to toxic buildup. Therefore, nutritional deficiencies can lead to back and joint pain. In addition, overeating augments the effect of hormones that support inflammation.

In their book *Myofascial Pain and Dysfunction*, Drs. Janet G. Travell and David G. Simons maintain that nearly half of the patients they treat suffering from chronic muscle and soft tissue pain have vitamin deficiencies.[11] But vitamins are only part of the story. In my practice, I found that most Americans are deficient in minerals and enzymes, as well—a situation that must be resolved before pain relief can be achieved.

Traditional Chinese Medicine (TCM) understands the importance of good nutrition in maintaining balance in the body and the flow of chi, or vital energy. In the Western approach to disease and pain, the main goal is to kill the bacteria (if any are present) and suppress the symptoms. The TCM approach is to reinforce the body and let it do the killing of the pathogens or fight the painful inflamed back. TCM seeks a way of eating that creates harmony and balance. TCM emphasizes not the disease, which already has developed, but the prevention of the disease. The emphasis should not be on back pain itself but on helping the body rid itself of the problem causing the back pain—the disharmony.

Therefore, an important step in regaining health is to achieve proper exercise, emotional balance, and proper nutrition to nourish the body, mind, and spirit. The ancient

Chinese were very much in tune with their bodies and their environment. They lived by the principle of existing in harmony with nature, and they maintained this balance in every segment of their lives—particularly in diet and nutrition.

Vitamin Deficiencies

Vitamins are organic, destructible nutrients required by the body in small amounts. Many vitamins (especially vitamin C and the B complex vitamins) play essential roles in normal body metabolism as coenzymes to a number of enzymes. Enzymes are substances naturally produced by the body that are required for normal metabolism, breathing, digestion— every phase of life. Coenzymes are helpers required by many enzymes for proper function. What this means is that some enzymes in your body cannot function at all without vitamins as part of their makeup. (See Table 4.1.)

Table 4.1

VITAMIN DEFICIENCIES AND BACK PAIN

VITAMIN	HOW A DEFICIENCY RELATES TO BACK PAIN
Vitamin A	A deficiency can cause painful joints. However, be aware that too much vitamin A is not a good thing, as it may cause a severe throbbing headache and joint or bone pain.
Thiamine (B_1)	A deficiency can lead to muscle wasting and weakness. Nerve processes depend heavily on vitamin B_1. It is most critical for synthesis of neurotransmitters and as an energy vitamin. Your need for this vitamin increases when you exercise.

(Continued)

Table 4.1 *(Continued)*

VITAMIN	HOW A DEFICIENCY RELATES TO BACK PAIN
Riboflavin *(B₂)*	A deficiency can cause nerve tissue damage.
Niacin *(B₃)*	A deficiency may interfere with nervous system health.
Biotin	A deficiency causes muscle pain, weakness, and fatigue.
Pyridoxine *(B₆)*	A deficiency can cause muscle twitching and may interfere with nerve transmission.
Folic acid	A deficiency of this vitamin can hinder DNA (deoxyribonucleic acid) synthesis, which is involved in protein syntheses.
Cobalamins *(forms of vitamin B₁₂)*	A deficiency interferes with protein synthesis and normal nerve transmission.
Vitamin C	A deficiency can cause muscle pain and degeneration, bone fragility, and joint pain.
Vitamin D	A deficiency of this vitamin can result in misshapen bones (because of faulty calcification) and muscle spasms.
Vitamin E	A deficiency can lead to loss of reflexes and muscle coordination, as well as neuromuscular dysfunction involving the spinal cord.

Mineral Deficiencies

Minerals perform a number of roles in the body. Certain minerals function as cofactors, inorganic components of enzyme systems that catalyze the metabolism of lipids, carbohydrates, and proteins. Some minerals act to regulate nerve and muscle function, while others provide rigidity to the skeleton or regulate electrolyte and fluid balance. Minerals also work together with hormones, peptides, vitamins, and other substances to regulate the body's metabolism.

Many minerals are necessary for enzymes to function. The mineral cofactors include calcium, cobalt, copper, iron, magnesium, manganese, molybdenum, phosphorus, potassium, selenium, silica, and zinc. (See Table 4.2.)

Table 4.2

MINERAL DEFICIENCIES AND BACK PAIN

MINERAL	HOW A DEFICIENCY RELATES TO BACK PAIN
Calcium	A deficiency can cause bone loss, especially osteoporosis, because calcium is the principal mineral of bones and teeth. Calcium is also involved in nerve function and muscle relaxation and contraction.
Iron	A deficiency can cause anemia, which interferes with oxygen transport to the cells.

(Continued)

Table 4.2 *(Continued)*

MINERAL	HOW A DEFICIENCY RELATES TO BACK PAIN
Magnesium	A deficiency of magnesium can cause weakness. This mineral is involved with calcium in bone mineralization and is required for normal muscle contraction and nerve impulse transmission.
Manganese	A deficiency of manganese can lead to nervous system disorders.
Phosphorus	A deficiency can interfere with bone and tooth formation, since phosphorus is a principal mineral of teeth and bones.
Potassium	One of the earliest symptoms of potassium deficiency is muscle weakness. This mineral plays an important role in muscle contraction and nerve transmission.
Selenium	A deficiency may lead to nervous system disorders.
Sodium	A deficiency may cause muscle cramps, since sodium is essential for muscle contraction and proper nerve transmission.
Zinc	A deficiency can interfere with proper function of more than 300 enzyme systems in the body that require zinc. A deficiency can also inhibit proper healing, since zinc plays an important role in wound healing.

Enzyme Deficiencies

Our bodies naturally produce and contain enzymes, substances responsible for everything that occurs in our body. At present, researchers have identified more than three thousand different kinds of enzymes in the human body—we've got millions of these things constantly renewing, maintaining, and protecting us. Every second of our lives, these enzymes are changing and renewing, sometimes at an unbelievable rate.

If we don't have enough enzymes, our body's ability to function, to repair when injured, and to ward off disease will be compromised. That's why an enzyme deficiency can be so devastating. Enzyme depletion can affect our endocrine system, including the pituitary gland, which regulates other glands, leading to excess weight, fatigue, and illness.

The reasons for enzyme depletion are many. Enzyme-dead diets, disease, chemotherapy, stress, physical injuries, illness, or digestive problems can all affect our enzyme levels. A decline in the body's production of enzymes interferes with the universal harmony within our body. When we reach a point where our body cannot produce certain enzymes, life will end.

There are a number of signs when we don't have enough enzymes. Probably the first sign is disturbed digestion. This is easily corrected by eating more whole foods or perhaps taking enzyme supplements.

But another sign of enzyme shortage that might not be so easy to recognize is free radical formation. Many researchers believe that we should live at least to the age of 120. However, the average American lives to age 70. Why does this happen? Because of the pollutants and free radicals in our environment, as well as the free radicals produced in our own body. Wrinkling is a sign of free radical formation (cross-linking). We can fight free radical damage with antioxidants (free radical scavengers). Several enzymes are antioxidants. Three of the best known are superoxide dismutase (SOD), catalase, and glutathione peroxidase. These enzymes fight free radicals that can destroy our bodies.

Why Are We Deficient in Important Nutrients?

Improper diets, increased demands, individual differences, and drug interactions all play a role in setting us up for vitamin, mineral, and enzyme deficiencies. In many cases, people just don't eat right and don't consume enough of a particular nutrient. Fast food is not known for its nutrient content. In fact, J. B. Cordaro, president of the Council for Responsible Nutrition, testified to the U.S. House of Representatives Subcommittee on Health and the Environment on July 29, 1993, that "unfortunately, most Americans do not get even the Recommended Dietary Allowance (RDA) of many nutrients from their normal diets. A national survey of over 21,000 people showed that not one of them received 100 percent of the RDA for ten basic nutrients from their diet alone."[12]

But even if you try to eat right, it is almost impossible to obtain nutrient-rich foods in today's society. Because of pesticides, preservatives, long storage times, and food-processing methods, many of the foods on your grocer's shelves no longer have the life-giving vitamins, minerals, and enzymes they had when they were first picked. Other foods are so highly processed or refined that there's very little nutritional value left. In addition, we're all different. What might be a proper diet for me may not provide enough nutrients for someone else. This is why supplements are so important.

Increased Demands

In many cases, injury and stress place increased nutrient demands on the body. The neuroendocrine responses and pain produced when tissues are injured are responsible for alterations in the nutritional requirements during and after accidental trauma or surgery and in the mechanisms of nutrition. Reflex responses and pain cause a loss or decrease of appetite, interfere with gastrointestinal activity, result in a marked delay of stomach emptying, increase the time it takes for food to pass through the colon, and increase nitrogen waste product buildup. Pain decreases appetite, and if severe enough, can result in nausea and even vomiting, thus interfering with the ability to eat.

RAPID REVIEW

- Back pain results from physical, emotional, and nutritional imbalances, or an overlapping of any or all of these factors, which can interfere with the flow of chi. In part 3 of this book, we will explain how to repair your body's imbalances, regain health, and fight back pain.

- Physical imbalances can be caused by injuries such as strains and sprains, poor posture, disk protrusions, congenital and developmental abnormalities, degenerative changes, pregnancy, muscular problems, gait irregularities, and lack of physical fitness. These and other physical problems usually involve some degree of inflammation that ultimately leads to back pain.

- Emotional imbalances set off a chain of physical responses in the body, typified by the fight-or-flight reaction. Emotional imbalance caused by stress can cause and perpetuate physical symptoms, including back pain.

- Nutritional imbalances and deficiencies can also interfere with proper bone formation and maintenance, muscle strength, and nervous system health. They can also lead to toxic buildup. All of these factors can cause and perpetuate back pain.

Five

Are Drugs Dangerous in the Treatment of Back Pain?

T o alleviate back pain, physicians in the United States usually prescribe nonsteroidal anti-inflammatory drugs (NSAIDs) such as aspirin, ibuprofen, or indomethacin; corticosteroids; muscle relaxants; painkillers; and antidepressants. In recent years, consumers have become increasingly concerned about the serious long-term side effects of these drugs. In addition, drugs can interfere with the flow of chi.

Although NSAIDs may work quickly to relieve inflammation, pain, and swelling, they can irritate the stomach if used for more than a few days. They can also cause microscopic bleeding that can lead to ulcers and other gastrointestinal problems. The effects of stronger prescription drugs can be even more devastating. For example, in up to 30 percent of patients, muscle relaxants cause drowsiness and, according to one report, may not be any more effective than NSAIDs in the treatment of back pain.[1] Opioid analgesics, which include morphine derivatives and synthetic drugs, are sometimes prescribed for pain relief. Although effective at masking the pain, they do nothing to cure the underlying problem. In addition, their side effects can be severe and may include drowsiness, altered judgment, and decreased reaction time. Nausea, impaired vision, constipation, and dizziness may also occur.[1] Antidepressants are sometimes used in the treatment of back pain, presumably because they may have some type of pain-relieving effect. The side effects of antidepressants can include drowsiness, constipation, dry mouth, urinary retention, and mania.[1]

The greatest amount of controversy seems to surround the use of corticosteroids, which have a long history of use in treating inflammation and pain. These drugs, which are given orally, epidurally, and intramuscularly, can cause serious, long-term side effects, including the following:

- *Decreased cortisone production within the body.* When cortisone is supplied from an outside source, the body learns that it doesn't need to make as much (or any) of this hormone—it's already getting enough from outside sources. But it takes time for the adrenal glands to resume production when the medication is suddenly stopped. Insufficient cortisone levels can leave the body unable to tolerate stress. An abrupt decline in cortisone levels in the blood can cause rapidly falling blood pressure, which can lead to shock and possibly death. Similar effects can result when cortisone creams or ointments are used for an extended time.[2]
- *Delayed healing.* Cortisone's action suppresses local inflammation, but it may actually delay healing.[3]
- *Progressive joint deterioration.* Cortisone and other steroids have a negative effect on collagen formation,[4] and progressive joint deterioration may occur with chronic use of cortisone.[5-7]
- *Skin changes,* including rashes and acne.
- *Spontaneous fractures* and other skeletal changes.
- *A loss of protein and calcium from bone,* especially when the dosage is prolonged or high.[8]
- *Central nervous system changes,* including psychotic changes.[9]

- *Metabolic changes*, including a decrease in carbohydrate tolerance (even in those with normal pretreatment tolerance)[8] and generalized obesity in some individuals (due to increased food intake).[10] The individual may develop a "moon face" (rounding of the facial contours) because of increased fat deposits in the cheeks. Less frequently, a "buffalo hump" can develop from fat deposits in the back of the neck.
- *Changes in electrolytic and water balance*, since cortisone can increase potassium excretion and lead to sodium retention, especially when taken in high doses.
- *Circulatory changes*, such as slight-to-significant blood pressure increase.
- *Gastrointestinal changes*, such as the worsening of gastric and duodenal ulcers (sometimes even leading to bleeding and perforation).[11]
- *Hormonal changes*, including a decrease in gonadal activity,[12] decreased libido, or irregular menses.
- *Eye problems*, such as the formation of cataracts or glaucoma.[13]
- *Decreased resistance to infections* (because of cortisone's immunosuppressive effect).
- *Avascular necrosis of bone* (when a bone dies and deteriorates because of lack of blood).[14,15]

DRUG INTERACTIONS

Not only do the drugs we take have serious side effects on our bodies, but they also can cause drug interactions, which then compound their dangerous side effects. Many people, especially those suffering from back pain, take many different prescription and over-the-counter (OTC) medicines that interfere with nutrient absorption or metabolism. Frequently, people take different drugs from different specialists for any number of conditions. The effect on the body can be devastating. Over-the-counter and prescription drugs can be a sharp two-edged sword. You may be taking drugs to relieve your back pain. However, the resulting nutritional deficiencies and side effects that can develop from these drugs might be worse than the condition itself. The following scenario could happen to any of us.

At seventy-five years of age, Margaret lives a drug-taking nightmare. Her cupboard is literally overflowing with bottles of various drugs. Margaret's plight is one we see all too frequently, particularly in the aging.

Margaret developed ulcers, so her doctor prescribed a stomach acid blocker. A rash soon appeared, followed by constipation, nausea, confusion, headaches, and fever. Her heart began to beat faster and irregularly. Margaret didn't know that antacids increase the demand for vitamin B_1 and that a deficiency of this vitamin can affect the heart, the gastrointestinal tract, the nervous system, and the general disposition. Antacids can also increase the demand for several minerals, including phosphorus, calcium, and iron.

Margaret returned to her doctor, who gave her additional drugs to treat her new symptoms. But the rash continued, so she visited her dermatologist, who promptly prescribed skin rash medicine.

In addition to her previous symptoms, Margaret developed a crushing sensation across her chest (possibly angina) and high blood pressure. Her arrhythmia not only persisted but became more severe. She saw a heart specialist for these symptoms and was given even more medicine. Margaret's stash of prescribed drugs was growing with every visit.

During this time, Margaret's husband of forty years died suddenly. She became extremely depressed and was given antidepressant medicine. She soon developed trouble breathing, chills, itching, a worse rash, anxiety, dizziness, ringing in the ears, fatigue, and headaches. She also began to gain weight, and her back started to hurt. She couldn't sleep and began to have thoughts of killing herself. Antidepressants can increase the demand for riboflavin (vitamin B_2). A deficiency of this important vitamin can result in nerve tissue damage, inflammation of the mucous membranes, dizziness, and dermatitis.

Margaret's joints began to ache, so her doctor recommended a nonsteroidal anti-inflammatory drug. NSAIDs can increase the need for vitamin C. As we know, these drugs not only have side effects but can greatly decrease the immune system's ability to fight off other diseases. From this drug, Margaret was "blessed" with swelling in her legs and arms, worsening headaches, blurred vision, ringing in the ears, stomach cramps, asthma, rash, nausea, and bronchospasms. To decrease the swelling, she was given a diuretic, which increased the demand for folic acid, vitamins B_2, B_6, and B_{12}, and several minerals, including potassium, calcium, magnesium, and zinc.

But Margaret is not alone. Many of us are not aware of the potential side effects of the drugs we take every day. And the older we get, the more pills we pop. The elderly are a prime target. Although they comprise only about 10 percent of the U.S. population, those over age sixty-five take about 25 percent of all the drugs prescribed and about the same proportion of OTC drugs.[16] So the rest of us are taking the remaining 75 percent of these drugs! We're drugstore druggies. Unfortunately, the majority of elderly people take two to five different drugs every day, which may be why they experience two to three times more adverse drug effects than do younger people.[17] The drugs they use most often are for constipation, cardiovascular disease, and conditions that affect the central nervous system. The most serious reactions are from cardiovascular and psychoactive drugs.[16] And because they take many of these drugs for long periods of time, older Americans are not as able to metabolize these drugs and are therefore more susceptible to serious, long-term side effects and the nutritional deficiencies these drugs can produce. But we don't have to be elderly to suffer nutritional deficiencies from the drugs we take. We all can be part of this unhappy group.

Like most of us, Margaret never questioned the care she was receiving. She grew up at a time when a physician's word was close to the word of God, when doctors made house calls, and when Drs. Kildare and Welby were paragons on TV, curing every sickness in twenty-six minutes plus commercials. Margaret believed the commercials. She believed that "miracle drugs" were here to save humankind. After all, weren't drug company researchers working night and day to cure everything from hangnails to the common cold?

Today, more than ever, we cannot afford to be like Margaret. We must take charge of our own lives. Turn to natural alternatives whenever possible. Remember, you cannot rely on others to keep you healthy. Your life is too precious. You must educate yourself and do all you can to stay healthy.

HOW DO DRUGS AFFECT US?

There are too many drugs with side effects to list them all here. Here is but a brief sample:

- Antibiotics can interfere with the absorption of carotene, vitamin A, and vitamin K and can increase the demand for folic acid, vitamins A, B_2, B_6, and B_{12}, and certain minerals, including calcium, iron, magnesium, and potassium.
- Anti-inflammatory drugs can increase the need for vitamins A, B_{12}, and C as well as potassium and can interfere with immune system function.
- Oral contraceptives can affect metabolic processes involving essential vitamins and minerals. Used by an estimated ten million women in the United States, they can increase the demand for vitamins (including A, B_2, B_6, B_{12}, C, and folic acid) and minerals (such as zinc and magnesium).
- Anticonvulsants can speed up the metabolism and elimination of vitamin D and can cause a folate deficiency.
- Alcohol (yes, it's a drug!) can interfere with the body's ability to absorb fats and proteins as well as the fat-soluble vitamins (A, D, E, and K).
- Antituberculars can increase the demand for vitamins (B_6, B_{12}, and folic acid) and minerals (calcium, magnesium, iron, and potassium).
- Drugs taken for hypertension can interfere with the metabolism of proteins, fats, and carbohydrates, resulting in glucose intolerance and hyperlipidemia, and increase the demand for vitamin B_6.
- Diuretics reduce the resorption by the kidneys of minerals such as potassium, thus increasing their excretion. Diuretics can also increase the demand for vitamins (B_2, B_6, B_{12}, and folic acid) and minerals (calcium, magnesium, potassium, and zinc).

WHAT CAN YOU DO?

What can you do to decrease the possibility of nutritional deficiencies and side effects caused by the drugs you take? Here are a few suggestions:

1. Take drugs only when absolutely necessary.
2. Get a second opinion whenever drugs are prescribed, and specifically ask about side effects and if the drug can cause any nutritional deficiencies.
3. List all your medications and make sure your physician has a copy of the list.
4. Stay healthy. Make sure you eat a well-balanced diet, including plenty of fresh vegetables and fruits. People who eat a poor diet are more susceptible to drugs and their side effects.
5. Take nutritional supplements, especially if you know that your drug depletes a particular nutrient. Review the importance of enzymes, minerals, and vitamins on your health and wellness.
6. Become more aware of what your drugs are doing to you and of drug interactions.
7. Don't be afraid to ask questions!

RAPID REVIEW

■ Cortisone and corticosteroids, NSAIDs, and multiple drugs are not the answer to back pain. They merely compound the problem and cause serious side effects.

■ Drugs and their metabolic by-products can cause toxic buildup, resulting in disharmony and interference with the flow of chi.

■ Use natural alternatives, including vitamins, minerals, enzymes, and herbs, whenever possible to improve the symptoms of back pain.

The Five-Step Jump-Start Plus Program in part 3 truly gives some light at the end of the aggravating back pain tunnel. Part 3 will begin to lay out the answers to pain relief.

Part Three

How to Cure Your Back Pain and Bring Harmony and Balance Back into Your Life

Six

The Triangle
of Health

W e're bombarded daily by physical, emotional, and nutritional stresses, any of which can disturb the body's harmony, interfere with the flow of chi, and lead to imbalances in body function. Identifying your stressors and other causes of body imbalance is only half the equation. Now that you know the possible causes and perpetuating factors for your back pain, what can you do about them?

Part 3 will show you how to restore your body balance, restore the flow of vital energy, and cure your back pain by using the Five-Step Jump-Start Plus Program. This is a rehabilitation program proven effective for optimizing health. It was born during my quest to rehabilitate my son David, honed through the long years of his return to health, and crystallized by successfully healing patients of all ages and occupations, including world-class athletes.

Always remember that the elimination or control of back pain and a return to wellness must involve your entire body. You must take steps to improve your emotional state, your physical health, and your nutritional status. Think of your health as a triangle. (See Figure 6.1.) Each side—physical, emotional, and nutritional—should be equal and in harmony with the others because each side is essential for the maintenance of health. If one side of the triangle is weak, it will lead

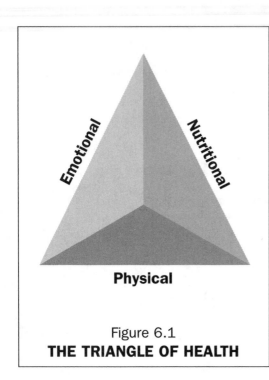

Figure 6.1
THE TRIANGLE OF HEALTH

to an imbalance in the body, causing the other sides to collapse. Illness and pain will result. For example, suboptimal nutrition will have profound effects on your emotional and physical health. At the same time, emotional stress can undermine any steps you take to improve your physical or nutritional status.

THE BODY'S INNATE ABILITY TO MAINTAIN HEALTH

Within your body is an innate potential to maintain health and overcome injury and illness. Each organism has mechanisms of self-repair. The process is present and active in every cell of the body, beginning with DNA—the macromolecules that define life and that act in each cell as mechanisms of self-repair. Your healing system is continuously on call and always operating, although not always as efficiently as needed. By energizing your body's self-healing mechanisms, you can eliminate pain and its underlying causes.

So how do you trigger your body's own ability to repair? Follow the steps outlined in this part of the book. They have been designed to allow and assist your body to help itself by restoring an innate balance, strengthening your body's inner defenses, and letting you fight pain, injury, and illness more effectively and efficiently, regardless of the cause.

My Five-Step Jump-Start Plus Program includes the following key areas involving all three sides of the triangle of health:

Emotional Health *(see chapter 7)*
Step 1: Positive mental attitude through mind and spirit power.

Nutritional Health *(see chapter 8)*

Step 2:   Detoxification

Step 3:   Diet

Step 4:   Supplements

Physical Health *(see chapter 9)*

Step 5:   Exercises (including tai chi chuan), plus Traditional Chinese Medicine and holistic techniques

THERAPY

There are some universals in the treatment of back pain:

- Do no harm to yourself.
- Balance your emotional state (see chapter 7).
- Improve your nutrition (see chapter 8):
  - Begin by including those therapies that help cleanse and detoxify the body, thus returning the whole body to balance. Treat those organs that are essential for detoxification and overall body performance, including the liver, kidneys, lungs, and spleen, as well as those that regulate bowel movements, improve circulation, and maintain immune function.
  - Eat a healthy diet.
  - Supplement with vitamins, minerals, enzymes, and other nutrients.
  - Use herbs to heal.
- Improve your body physically through exercises and TCM/holistic techniques (see chapter 9).

FACTORS AFFECTING YOUR RECOVERY TIME

The amount of time needed to recover from your back condition will vary, depending on a number of factors:

- The duration of your symptoms. The longer you have had the symptoms, the longer it will take for you to return to normal. In one study, 85 percent of those patients treated within seven days of the onset of pain were cured within six months.[1] By contrast, only 35 percent of patients were cured when treatment began more than twenty-eight days after the onset of pain.

- The severity of any trauma.
- The intensity of your pain.
- The number of similar prior episodes.
- Your lifestyle.
- Your health at the time you first experienced back pain.
- Your weight.
- Your age.
- Your occupation.
- Your attitude.
- Your genetics.
- The degree to which you cooperate and participate in your own healing.

A NOTE ABOUT SURGERY

There are times when surgery is mandatory, such as in the case of a severely herniated disk. However, you should only consider surgery as a last resort. It's interesting to note that in the United States, twice as many people have surgery for low back pain than do people in most other developed countries.[2] Just think about that!

Developing a healthy lifestyle by implementing my Five-Step Jump-Start Plus Program can greatly improve your body's reaction to the physical, emotional, and nutritional stressors affecting you every day. It can help you return your body to a healthy balance and to optimal health and restore the flow of vital energy (chi). The following chapters will explain how to implement each part of the plan.

Note: One should always consult a physician before beginning a program of self-treatment.

Seven

Mind and Spirit Power: Returning to Emotional Harmony

Back pain can be the result of many interacting factors. Although you may have a physical problem causing your back pain, you may also have experienced an emotionally traumatic event—a difficult divorce, the death of a loved one, stress at work, or some other emotionally charged life crisis. Such factors can actually worsen and perpetuate your back pain because they throw your emotional harmony out of balance, affecting your entire body.

Mental stress can be a major cause of back pain. Understanding and accepting this concept is important. As the Bible says in Romans 12:2, "Be ye transformed by the renewing of your mind." To heal yourself, you must regain your emotional balance.

Many people complain of emotional stress. It can worm its way into every aspect of your existence, interfering with your enjoyment of life and even keeping you from sleeping.

Judging by the number of sleeping pills sold every year in the United States, stress must interfere with a lot of sleep! But drugs aren't the answer. Stress reduction is.

My father was a wonder. Although he was under great pressure every day from work, he slept like a log and woke up refreshed and ready for another day. He did not listen to the news before retiring. He didn't drink a nightly cup of coffee or ingest any other stimulants before going to bed. However, he did take a fifteen- to thirty-minute walk and he knelt and prayed every night before climbing into bed. I know that the walk in the fresh air was good physical exercise and gave him a chance to unwind. The prayers were a form of meditation. They filled his mind with peaceful and positive thoughts and allowed him to gain and accept mental peace.

CONTROLLING EMOTIONAL STRESS

How can you control the emotional stress in your life? The first step is to identify the factors causing the stress. This may not be as easy as it sounds. Does the nightly news worry you? How do you react when your favorite team makes a stupid error and loses the game? Do these and other events cause you stress? If so, you need to put things in perspective. This is very obvious, but it must be stated: There are certain things you can control in life and other things over which you have no control, like the weather, or the daily workings of the government, or what your team does out on the field. When you learn to recognize the difference between what you can and cannot control, you will find that your stress level decreases enormously.

Keeping a diary is a good way to discover what is causing you stress and to what degree. Whenever a stressful event occurs, take note of the following:

- What happened?
- When and where did it happen?
- What made it a stressful event?
- How did you respond to the event?
- Was your response appropriate to the event? If not, why not? Did you overreact?

After several days, perhaps weeks, you can analyze your diary and begin to see a pattern as to how, when, and why you react to certain events. This will help you learn to recognize and control your stress.

Also listen to your body for clues. If you feel your neck and shoulder muscles tensing or you feel a headache coming on every time you sit down with your supervisor, you're probably under stress. If you grind your teeth or feel like flying into a rage, you need to implement the following steps to attain a positive mental attitude: part 1 of the Five-Step Jump-Start Plus Program.

STEPS TO LIVING A STRESS-FREE LIFE
- Identify what causes stress in your life. Change the things that you can change and learn to accept the rest.
- Take a "time out" whenever stress starts to pile up. Take a few minutes every morning and evening to practice deep breathing, meditation, or other relaxation techniques.
- Avoid frustrations. If traffic congestion makes you hyper, plan to avoid it by leaving earlier or later than normal. Relaxing music or inspirational tapes can also help.
- If nothing seems to work, consider professional counseling.

POSITIVE MENTAL ATTITUDE
A positive mental attitude (PMA) is an attitude adjustment or "nutrition of the mind," as Joan Priestley, M.D., calls it.[1] Dr. Priestley is a world-famous researcher, writer, and speaker on the treatment of HIV/AIDS. She has used PMA extensively in her treatment of AIDS patients. PMA can help you achieve stress reduction by putting a positive spin on life through relaxation, deep breathing, meditation, biofeedback, autogenics (autosuggestion, or mind over matter), progressive muscle relaxation exercises, and visualization. Dr. Priestley adds, "Many people carry around a lot of emotional baggage" that must be eliminated before they can overcome back pain. PMA can help you do this.

Unfortunately, it may be difficult to keep a positive mental attitude because back pain can be very frustrating and depressing. Sometimes a negative attitude can cause us to be our own worst enemy. We may make very hurtful statements that can drive even our closest friends away. At a time when we desperately need encouragement and love, we can isolate ourselves from others.

Making our attitude even worse may be the fact that enjoyable sex may become more difficult, if not impossible, because of back pain. The more severe and debilitating the cause of back pain, the longer the recovery time and the greater the possibilities of divorce (if married) or severance of meaningful relationships.

A negative attitude can be a major problem. But in a few short weeks, it is possible to become confident and regain the positive mental attitude you had as a child, back when anything was possible. Approach both life and the relief of back pain with a positive mental attitude—with the conviction that even the elimination of your back pain is possible. Dare to think positively and you will find life's challenges to be enjoyable experiences rather than stressful events.

Jack is a great example of the effect that a positive mental attitude can have on your life. Jack had polio when he was a child and walked with a decided limp because his left leg was more than 1 inch shorter than his right. This imbalance caused considerable hip and leg pain. Jack used crutches and walked stiff-legged because of restrictive braces. Running was a challenge because his legs and crutches seemed to want to flail in all directions. As Jack grew, he was fitted with sole and heel lifts in his shoes to help balance his leg length.

Jack was determined to walk like a normal child. Although he stumbled and often fell, he got right up again and kept trying. He often had bloody knees and torn pants, but he kept plugging away.

Eventually, Jack learned to walk without crutches and then to run. He ran everywhere—to downtown Davenport, to school, or to the store, always with a slight limp but with a smile on his face. His wiry spindle legs pumped like two pile-driving pistons. When Jack entered college, he decided—as illogical as it sounds—to play football. The long years on crutches had strengthened his now anvil-like arms and hands. The football stuck to his fingers as though it were glued. Jack ran like the wind, short leg, limp, and all.

Although his coach was reluctant to use a player with Jack's physical limitations, Jack persevered and proved he could do it. Not only did he play football for St. Ambrose College, he became a small-college All-American end. He subsequently served in combat in World War II and was in the Battle of the Bulge at a time when people with physical limitations were routinely barred from entry into the U.S. Army.

Despite seemingly insurmountable odds, Jack overcame many obstacles in his life by setting and achieving goals through commitment and a belief that he could succeed. This man never gave up and never let a physical impairment keep him from being a champion. If Jack could do it, so can you.

HOW TO HAVE A POSITIVE MENTAL ATTITUDE

- Learn to relax.
- Think thoughts and use words that are positive, motivating, and encouraging. Tell yourself over and over again that you can do it—no matter what "it" is.
- Envision your success. "What the mind conceives, the body achieves."
- Never give up—keep on keeping on. Each day you will improve.
- Learn to release pent-up anger and eliminate negative thoughts. Unexpressed emotions, particularly anger, can cause increased muscle tension and chronic back pain.
- Never call yourself or others a failure, nuts, crazy, ugly, stupid, or fat. Try not to label or prejudge yourself or others.
- Don't blame yourself or others when you make a mistake. Instead, try to think positively, learn from mistakes, and learn to prevent them before they occur.
- Imagine pain flowing out from your body.
- Learn to identify those things in life that you can control and those that you can't. Concentrate on the things you can change and ignore the rest.

RELAXATION

Relaxation is the first step in achieving a positive mental attitude, in controlling stress, and in balancing your body. If you feel tense, your muscles are tense. Tense muscles hurt and can affect the way you move. This, in turn, can cause muscular imbalance, leading to tension and pain elsewhere in the body. Sleep, of course, is the ultimate form of relaxation. It gives your tissues time to rebuild and your body and mind time to recharge.

There are many techniques that can help you balance the scale between relaxation and stress. No one technique is better than another, and what works for your neighbor might not work for you. Find the techniques that work best for you, your body, and your back and practice them daily.

Some of the best-known relaxation techniques include deep breathing exercises, meditation, biofeedback, visualization/conceptualization, and exercise.

Deep Conscious Breathing

One of the body's first responses to stress is shallow and rapid breathing. Relaxed, slow, and deep breathing is a wonderful way to turn off the stressor switch and begin to relax.

Everyone knows that breathing is essential for life and that without air we would die. We can live weeks without food, days without water, but only a few minutes without air. Unfortunately, as the body ages and is subjected to illness, injury, stress, or general wear and tear, we progress from deep abdominal breathing to shallow chest breathing. Our breaths become shorter and shallower. This means that with each breath, we may not be getting a sufficient quantity of oxygen to the cells in our body.

Observe a healthy infant, deep breathing from the abdomen. We must relearn how to breathe—something babies know instinctively. In this way, air—with its life-energizing oxygen—can better enter the body and flow to every cell. Deep breathing also creates a sense of relaxation and helps you eliminate stress.

HOW TO BREATHE EFFECTIVELY

- Practice breathing in a warm, quiet area free from noise and distractions.
- Wear comfortable, loose clothing.
- Never practice just after eating. Instead, practice between meals (at least one and a half to two hours before or after a meal).
- Sit or lie comfortably. If lying on the floor, lie on a blanket or a pad.
- Rest your hands on your stomach and relax. Let your body sink deeper and deeper into the warm earth.
- Inhale deeply through your nose. As you inhale, feel the tension collecting. Let the air pass through to the depths of your body. Let the breath sweep your mind as clear as the deep blue sky and leave your body as light as the clouds that occasionally pass by.
- Allow your stomach to expand to its maximum (do not tighten the stomach muscles). Your stomach will force your hands out if you are breathing properly.
- Hold your breath for a few seconds.
- Slowly exhale the air through your mouth. As you exhale, imagine the stress flowing out from your body. Separate your lips slightly and purse them as though you are preparing to whistle. This controls the speed at which air passes.
- Feel your stomach deflating as you exhale.
- Feel the natural rise and fall of your stomach.
- Feel a deeper sense of relaxation each time you exhale.
- Feel your arms relaxing, your legs relaxing, your neck, face, and shoulders relaxing.
- A calmness comes over your whole being. Feel your body sinking even deeper and the peaceful calm spreading over you like a warm, soft breeze. With each deep breath and exhalation, you can feel the stress and disharmony leaving your body and peace returning.
- Repeat the inhalation/exhalation cycle at least four or five times during each session.
- Practice deep breathing for a few minutes at least two or three times every day and whenever you begin to feel tense and stressed.

Meditation

Another good way to relax is through the ancient discipline of meditation. "Meditation is the art of suspending verbal and symbolic thinking for a time, somewhat as a courteous audience will stop talking when a concert is about to begin," says Alan Watts, credited with introducing meditation to the West.[2] Meditation can help you to achieve total relaxation and discover your inner being. Some people feel that meditation enriches the blood with life-giving oxygen. It is a way to discover yourself and put your life in perspective. Meditation helps to free the health-giving energy from within your body and to release deadly toxins, which drain your vitality. Meditation decreases stress, clears your mind of cobwebs, and allows your body to work at an optimal level.

Yoga, Tai Chi, and Qi Gong

Yoga, tai chi, and qi gong exercises are a marriage of body, mind, and spirit. However, because these exercises are primarily physical, as well as meditative, they are described in chapter 9, "Physical Healing Secrets." These exercises should be used in conjunction with the techniques explained in this chapter. Remember, just as a river is made of many individual drops of water, so does your back treatment program involve many different techniques and the daily use of these proven techniques. Repeating daily is the secret to the program's success.

Biofeedback

Biofeedback is an effective way to identify and learn to control the stressors in your life. In this technique, instruments record biological functions (the *bio* in *biofeedback*). Biological functions include the tension in your muscles, which can be measured by electrical impulses from contracting muscles, and the warmth of your skin, which can be measured using a thermometer. The feedback involves either a sound (which increases in pitch) or visual displays (such as changing colors or dials) that alert you when your muscles tense, your skin's temperature drops (which occurs as adrenaline diverts blood from the surface of your body to the core

KEYS TO MEDITATION

- Eliminate any possible distractions, such as ringing telephones or other noisy interruptions. However, an audiotape of ocean waves or of a rippling brook may actually be helpful.
- Remove your shoes and remove or loosen tight clothing.
- Sit comfortably or lie on a mat with a towel rolled up under your neck and another one under your knees. Allow your arms and hands to rest on your lap.
- Close your eyes, let your jaw relax, and take a deep breath. Slowly exhale, letting the air pass between your relaxed lips and partially separated teeth while slowly uttering the word *peace*, drawing out the vowel sounds "pe-e-e-a-a-c-c-c-e." Mentally focusing on a word (such as *peace*, *God*, or *one*) or on a pleasant image such as a beautiful, warm beach can be helpful.
- Continue to relax, breathe deeply, and focus mentally. Let your worries float away like clouds in a soft, pleasant breeze. Clear your mind and find a safe physical and mental retreat from all the stresses of the outside world.
- Feel the muscle tension in your head and neck gradually slip away. Then feel your shoulders and then your arms, hands, and fingers relax. You feel an inner calm flowing down through your legs, feet, and toes. Your chest and back relax. Finally, your entire body relaxes.
- As you gently come out of your meditation, inhale, exhale, relax, and stretch.
- Set aside ten, twenty, or thirty minutes every day to meditate and recharge your batteries.

in preparation for the fight-or-flight response), or when you begin to sweat (you sweat more when you are under stress). This feedback lets you know when your body is tensing and also gives you an effective way to measure the efficacy of any relaxation technique.

Biofeedback doesn't work for everyone. In fact, the older we get, the more difficult it is to change our ways. But biofeedback can be an efficient way to learn how to change physical reactions to stress because it is usually necessary for only a few weeks. However, it works better for some conditions than for others. It seems most successful in treating neck and upper back pain, migraines, and tension headaches. It is less successful with lower back pain.

Your physician can provide biofeedback instruments and explain how to use them.

Autogenics

Autogenics (or autosuggestion) is another method of relaxation. This technique is literally about placing mind over matter. Autosuggestion is accomplished by giving yourself certain mental clues. By doing this, you can tell your body how to produce a relaxation response and how to feel whenever it experiences stress or feels tense. This technique requires focus, time, practice, and commitment, but it has been used successfully for years in pain clinics and for various chronic disorders.

Autogenics is an extremely powerful technique. Athletes using this technique as part of a training program have broken national and world records.

Visualization: What the Mind Conceives, the Body Achieves

Visualization (also called conceptualization) is a way to actually visualize your body as it improves, healing itself through the activation of your own innate healing processes. Visualization can help decrease back pain and eliminate stress. By repeatedly visualizing a sequence of events where back pain is decreased, it is possible, little by little, to program yourself to expect and internalize a reduction in back pain. That is, what the mind conceives, the body achieves.

Visualization Exercises for Back Pain Visualize yourself living each day without back pain. Begin by imagining an entire day pain free (from the time you wake up in the morning until you go to bed at night). Visualize yourself going through the various activities of each day. Each time you confront a situation that would usually be stressful, imagine that you are able

AUTOGENICS TECHNIQUE

- Sit or lie comfortably. Any tight-fitting clothing should be loosened.
- Clear your mind of all distractions.
- Take a few deep breaths (inhale through the nose and exhale through the mouth). With the mouth slightly ajar, say "peace," "I feel at peace," "I am quiet," "My mind is restful," or similar statements.
- Mentally concentrate on your right arm and repeat to yourself, "My right arm feels heavy and warm."
- Then repeat a similar statement concentrating on your left arm, then your right leg, left leg, and so on, until you feel that all the stress is gone and you are fully relaxed.
- Take a deep breath and stretch as you complete the exercise. Exhale very slowly, open your eyes, and note how your body feels.
- Practice this technique at least twice a day for ten to fifteen minutes and whenever you are under stress. The more you do it, the easier it will become, and you will be able to relax your body, your back, and your mind in less time and with minimal effort.

to handle the difficult situation or the problem by practicing good coping skills, such as deep breathing and repeating to yourself over and over, "I am safe, I am protected." See yourself safe and cared for. See yourself performing in a powerful, healthy way and drawing from the inner energy, strength, power, and health that already exist within your body.

The people that walk on hot coals or sharp nails practice visualization to accomplish what they do. Further, Buddhist monks can lower their pulse rate using visualization and meditation. This technique is also frequently used by athletes as a key part of competition and an effective way to reach their goals.

I once worked with a world-class swimmer on visualization. His goal was to break the U.S. high school record for the 100-yard breaststroke. He learned to see himself during each stroke, the number of strokes needed for each length, and his final times. He conceptualized finishing at a specific time and what it felt like to set the U.S. high school record. The day of the state finals progressed as though we had written the script. He won the state championship, set the U.S. high school record, and was within one one-thousandth of a second of what we had projected as his competitive time. Unfortunately, we later learned that he had missed the world record by one one-hundredth of a second. Who knows? If we had been aware of the world record during his training, perhaps he could have slightly lowered his conceptualized time and set a world record! This is the power of visualization. What the mind conceives, the body achieves.

Visualization can help you control what you do. The doctors with the East German Olympic swim team (during its domination of Olympic sports) wanted to measure the swimmers' blood parameters while the athletes were at rest, after swimming 65 percent of maximum speed, and after swimming 85 percent of maximum speed. They needed this information to determine at what point during exercise the muscles were beginning to break down rather than build up. The athletes were told to swim at 65 percent of their fastest speed and then, after a break, to swim at 85 percent of their maximum speed. The athletes were able to accurately do this even without any mechanism to tell them how fast they were swimming. The innate mechanism in their bodies was subconsciously giving them instructions. They visualized their swim times and then just did it.

For your back, your health, and your life to improve, you must visualize that they are improving. The process works. To visualize your back pain diminishing and finally disappearing, try the following visualization voyage.

Relaxation Exercises

By performing relaxation exercises on a regular basis, you can give your body, mind, and spirit a chance to unwind and successfully prepare for the next stressful onslaught. Many people don't know how to relax and can't focus on relaxing. You may be so stressed that you don't even know the difference between relaxation and tension. The progressive muscle relaxation technique can help you to identify your tense muscles.

VISUALIZATION TECHNIQUE

- Sit comfortably or lie on a mat with a towel rolled up under your neck and another one under your knees. Allow your arms and hands to rest on your lap.
- Visualize that the waste products trapped in the tissue fluid of all your cells in the injured area are leaving and flowing back into the capillaries, through the bloodstream, and then leaving the body.
- Visualize the capillary walls rebuilding and repairing.
- Visualize nutrition and oxygen flowing to the injured area and beginning to repair the body.
- You can feel your body healing, the pain diminishing, and normal function returning.
- Practice visualization for ten to twenty minutes every day.

Progressive Muscle Relaxation Technique I first learned of this tension reliever when my wife, Margie, was pregnant with our first child, Tony. The birth preparation classes we attended taught Margie how to relax during labor. But you don't have to be pregnant to use this exercise. In fact, I have used this technique many times to effectively relax when muscle tension is on the attack. This technique will work for one or all of the muscle groups in your body.

- Consciously tense and then relax each segment of your body beginning with the muscles in the toes and then your feet. By first tensing the muscles in this way, you will have a way to gauge the muscle's initial tension. You may be surprised at how tense some of your muscles are.
- Continue tensing, then relaxing your muscles, working your way up your legs and thighs, across your abdomen, then your lower back, midback, fingertips, arms, shoulders, neck, jaw, and finally the scalp.
- This technique will get easier each time you practice. Usually, relaxation takes about ten to twenty minutes, but don't force yourself.

Back Muscle Relaxation Technique The following technique is an adaptation of the general principles we have just discussed, but relating specifically to back pain. This technique can be used anywhere—at your workstation, at home, while playing sports, or while driving. You can also combine this exercise with visualization techniques.

- Sit, lie, or stand in a relaxed position.
- Tighten the back muscles you want to target (upper back, midback, lower back).
- Note how it feels when the muscles are tight.
- Relax and release. Note how it feels to relax the muscles.
- Compare the difference. This helps to improve body awareness and to experience how relaxed muscles feel.

Back Alignment Relaxation Exercise This exercise can help relax your back and can also help to align your spine.

- Lie on the floor on your back.
- Place a rolled-up towel under your neck. Then either place two pillows under your knees or place your calves up on the seat of a chair (this position relieves stress on the lower back).
- Use this posture for meditation.
- Relax in this position for five to twenty minutes every day. *Note:* The legs and knees should be relaxed.

REINFORCEMENT

The success of your back pain rehabilitation is directly related to your own motivation. For you to succeed, reinforcement must be increased and maintained, both from within yourself and from others. Place a sign saying "I am special" or "I can do it" on your dresser, refrigerator, or anywhere you're likely to see it every day.

In a study reported in the *Journal of Counseling Psychology*, Professor Elisabeth M. Altmaier and associates stated that self-motivation is important during back pain treatment.[3] Individuals who received reinforcement reported less pain and improved function at follow-up assessments. Positive verbal reinforcement, persuasion, and rewards for accomplishments are beneficial in healing anyone with chronic lower back pain. If an individual has a nonsupportive or neglectful family, fewer gains can be made in the treatment of back pain.

SEXUAL FUNCTION

As with all natural phenomena, human sexuality is approached by the Chinese with a blend of reverence and curiosity. According to Daniel P. Reid, author of *The Tao of Health, Sex, and Longevity,*[4] the Chinese feel that sex is essential for overall health, balance, and well-being. However, the pleasure of sex can be diminished because of increased back pain, irritation, and discomfort during sex.

Energy and sexual essence are important tools to decreasing stress on the spiritual pathway to peace and bliss in life. How devastating, then, when this joy of sex becomes an exercise in pain. Sex is an important part of adult life, but physical impairment and back pain can greatly interfere with the joy, relaxation, and satisfaction of sex.

Back pain can have a definite effect on sexual function. In one study, Dr. Charles Vander Kolk and his associates demonstrated a 72 percent reduction in sexual functioning after back injury.[5] The greatest reduction was in surgical patients. The decrease in sex function was equal for both men and women. Therefore, for those with back pain, sex function and pleasure are decreased.

Human sexuality is as basic to human life as sleeping and eating. Since a healthy sex life is important to the overall wellness of the individual, alternative techniques and positions should be explored. Finding the best position for you and your partner is extremely important. Further, adopting different positions during intercourse exercises various joints and muscles, as well as stimulating different parts of your body. Different positions can suit various body types and physiques—and even those with back problems.

There are four fundamental positions for women and men during intercourse. The purpose of the different positions is to give the man and woman options so that their acts of sexual intercourse are physically and emotionally more pleasurable. Each position has many variations. The four fundamental sexual postures are (1) man on top, (2) woman on top, (3) side by side, face to face, and (4) man behind woman. If one position increases your back pain, try another one until you find what's best for you.

1. *Man on top*. In this position, the man lies on top of the woman or kneels between her thighs.
2. *Woman on top*. The man lies on his back, and the woman straddles the man's thighs. The woman controls the action in this position.
3. *Side by side, face to face*. In this position, the woman and man lie side by side, facing each other, and take various positions of entry. For both partners, this position is least tiring, but it requires coordination and some agility. It can best be used by individuals who are familiar with each other's responses.
4. *Man behind woman*. In this position, the woman crouches in front of the man on her knees, and the man kneels behind the woman. Another position is for the woman to lie on her stomach as the man lies behind her on his side.

These four basic Taoist postures can be modified. According to Taoist texts, there are "nine ways" and "thirty styles" or variations of sexual postures. Each individual with back pain can choose the position that works best for him or her.

RAPID REVIEW

There are a number of techniques to help you fight emotional stress, gain a positive mental attitude, and return your emotional status to a healthy balance. Although some stress is unavoidable—and life would be pretty boring without it—learn to keep stress in balance. Try to gain a positive mental attitude.

- Some people find meditation or visualization can keep them in a relaxed state. Others try deep breathing or other relaxation exercises.
- Breathing exercises, relaxation techniques, and meditation are excellent tools when used with yoga, qi gong, and tai chi exercises. These exercises are explained in chapter 10.
- No one technique is better than another. Experiment with all of them, and find the technique that works best for you.

Eight

Nutritional Power

Emotional, physical, and nutritional stress are like three overlapping circles, each affecting the other two and disturbing your body's overall balance. Normalizing all three is critical for optimal rehabilitation and wellness. This chapter will show you how to fight nutritional stress, which can cause imbalances that may perpetuate or even cause your back pain. (See Figure 8.1.)

To function properly, your body needs *macronutrients*, such as protein, carbohydrates, and fats, as well as *micronutrients*, including vitamins, minerals, and enzymes. A shortage of one or an excess of another can cause an imbalance in the body. This imbalance stresses the entire body. As mentioned in chapter 4, stress and body imbalance of any kind can set off a chain of physical responses that increase muscle tension and lead to spasms, organ dysfunction, and pain. Stress can also interfere with the absorption and utilization of

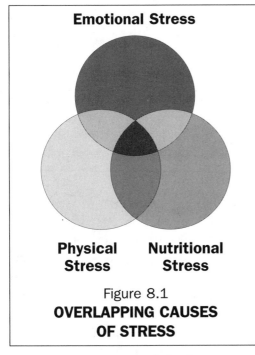

Emotional Stress

Physical Stress   **Nutritional Stress**

Figure 8.1
OVERLAPPING CAUSES OF STRESS

nutrients required for proper bone formation and nerve function. Improving your diet and increasing the intake of a few specific vitamins, minerals, enzymes, and other supplements can go a long way toward improving your body's overall health, as well as improving the function of muscles, tendons, ligaments; strengthening bones and organs; and reducing pain.

Traditional Chinese Medicine's view of nutrition is based on the principles of harmony and balance and direct knowledge of the nature of individual foods. TCM's view of nutrition has its roots in knowledge that is over six thousand years old. Longevity and health will be greatly improved for any person who studies, learns, and uses this time-tested, ancient knowledge.

TCM demands harmony and balance in your diet. In treating back pain, a doctor of TCM would first ask you to eat certain foods. He or she would look for an extreme imbalance in the energies found in the foods you currently eat or for a critical deficiency in vital nutrition.

Improving your body's biochemistry through better nutrition is also an important part of the Five-Step Jump-Start Plus Program and involves three steps, all of which are covered in this chapter:

1. Detoxification
2. Diet
3. Supplements

DETOXIFICATION

You probably have the oil changed periodically in your car to keep it mechanically tuned and running efficiently. Your body is like an engine in that it also requires periodic cleansing and removal of toxins. Detoxification through juice fasting, improved elimination, and increased water consumption is very important, even vital, to wellness and the elimination of back pain.

The first step in improving your nutritional profile is to eliminate toxins that have accumulated in your body. Toxins are harmful substances that can develop from the external environment or be produced from within the body. External toxins include alcohol, drugs, tobacco, microbial toxins, heavy metals, pesticides, solvents, and radiation. These and other foreign substances and pollutants continuously subject our body to increased stress. In addition, our modern lifestyle and unhealthy eating habits (including the excessive intake of fats and refined carbohydrates) can encourage the accumulation of toxins in our body.

In contrast to externally derived toxins, internal toxins can originate within us when the body's ability to rid itself of metabolic waste products breaks down. These metabolic wastes are created every minute of every day as our body processes the food, water, and air that we require for life. A good example is the way the body digests and metabolizes protein. Acids and enzymes secreted in the stomach break down the protein we eat, converting it into short chains of amino acids (protein is made up of about twenty common amino acids). These amino acids are further degraded in a process called *deamination*. One of the by-products of deamination is ammonia. You may be familiar with cleaning solutions containing ammonia—a strong-smelling, toxic compound. Ammonia is also a base (rather than an acid), so excessive production by the body will throw off the body's delicate acid-base balance. Therefore, it is important for the body to eliminate this toxic waste. To do this, the liver combines ammonia with carbon dioxide to form *urea*, which is much less toxic. Urea is then released into the blood, where it circulates through the kidneys and is eventually excreted in the urine. However, if the liver or kidneys are not functioning correctly, the toxic by-products cannot be properly eliminated from the body. Toxins can also be generated when nutrition is inadequate, when we are suffering from a disease, or if tissue oxidation is incomplete.

In addition to the roles played by the liver and kidneys, we continually excrete large quantities of wastes, toxins, and dangerous metabolic products through our lungs, intestines, and skin. The body strives to maintain good blood flow and lymphatic circulation at all times to facilitate this process. Blood not only carries oxygen and nutrients throughout the body to maintain cell metabolism but also cleans out the cells. It transports and eliminates metabolic debris and waste products.

Unfortunately, when our body's self-healing powers are overtaxed by toxins (whether external, internal, or both), it leads to stress on the body. This, in turn, can lead to organ imbalance (or dysfunction) and chronic degenerative disorders, including back problems and back pain. Our job, then, is to help the body help itself.

Step 1

Eliminate your exposure to external toxins. Buy organically grown food to avoid the possibility of pesticides, preservatives, and other additives; stop smoking; avoid alcohol and caffeine; and avoid polluted air and water as much as possible. See the Five-Step Jump-Start Plus Program's Dietary Do's and Don'ts on pages 100–101.

Step 2

Help your body rid itself of toxins by improving the body's own detoxification system. This can be achieved by improving the body's excretion mechanism through a properly functioning intestinal tract, by juice fasting, and by increasing your water intake.

It is especially important to keep the colon clean and free of debris. Sluggish intestinal function, including constipation, places tremendous stress on the body and allows toxins from food putrefaction to sit for long periods in the colon, where they are reabsorbed into the overburdened bloodstream and taken to the already overworked liver. See below for tips on how to avoid this condition.

CONSTIPATION

Constipation is a symptom, not a disease. It is characterized by an increase in stool hardness, a decrease in the frequency of defecation, or a difficulty in passing fecal matter. Rather than turning to harsh and sometimes harmful laxative drugs, try natural remedies:

- Drink plenty of fluids (eight to twelve glasses of water every day). Inadequate fluid consumption is a frequent cause of constipation.

- Increase your intake of fiber-rich foods, including fresh fruits and vegetables and whole grain cereals and breads. Fiber drinks such as Metamucil are also beneficial.
- Take digestive enzymes to help your body break down the foods you eat. Enzymes, such as proteases (which break up protein), lipases (which break up fats and cholesterol), and amylases (which break up starch and sugar), are essential to proper elimination. Ideally, these enzymes should be taken thirty minutes before eating, but you can take them just before or even with your meals. Effective amounts can vary, depending on the individual; follow instructions on the label. Gradually increase the dosage until loose bowels occur; then decrease the dose slightly.
- High doses of vitamin C appear to loosen the fecal matter in the large intestine and facilitate the evacuation of waste. However, increased vitamin C intake may actually cause loose bowels or diarrhea, so be sure to also increase your fluid intake.
- A number of herbs can help elimination, including cascara sagrada, flaxseed, psyllium seeds (used in many over-the-counter fiber products), senna, and rhubarb. Your local health food store probably has many natural herbal products. Follow the instructions on the label.
- Increase your intake of probiotics, including *Lactobacillus acidophilus, Lactobacillus bulgaricus,* and bifidobacteria (including *Bifidobacterium bifidum* and *Bifidobacterium longum*). Probiotics assist the beneficial bacteria in the colon (which are essential to proper digestive tract function) and may reduce the generation of toxic compounds produced in the intestinal tract. For best results, follow the instructions on the label.

Fasting

Therapeutic fasting has always been an important part of Taoist training programs and is one of the world's most natural and ancient healing mechanisms. As a means to detoxify the body, improve health, and increase longevity, fasting has been a way of life for centuries—be it along the Amazon or in Asia, central Africa, or ancient Greece.

In the tenth century A.D., Chang Tsung-cheng, physician for the Sung dynasty, wrote frequently on the therapeutic benefits of cleansing accumulated poisons and debris from the colon. He recommended colon cleanses for constipation; indigestion; aching, painful, and stiff joints; and emotional disturbances. Chang Tsung-cheng believed that a blocked stomach and bowels could result in energy and blood stagnation.

Waste accumulates in your body throughout your entire life. The older your body and the more you have stuffed it with "garbage," the greater the toxin saturation. Toxins can also be generated when the body suffers from pain. These toxins are swept from the body during a fast. Fasting quickly increases the elimination of body wastes and can augment the body's healing processes. It provides a physiological vacation for the body's organs and glands. For this reason, fasting is extremely valuable in fighting chronic disease. The regeneration of tissues and the purification of the body as a whole restores youthful vigor to the body. Fasting and colon cleansing relieves your body of metabolic waste products, pollutants, toxins, and unwanted microbes. It gives your gastrointestinal tract a spring cleaning, relieving stress on the kidneys, lungs, colon, blood, and immune system.

Fasting is necessary for longer life because it eliminates body disharmony. For example, when there is acid buildup in the bloodstream, acid crystals can deposit in the joints, causing joint and back pain. Where spurs are formed, this actually fuses the joints together (for example, ankylosing spondylitis, or "bamboo spine"). The result is pain and disability. By fasting, your body's own nutrients can enter the joints and break up the crystals, resulting in improved joint function, improved joint mobility, and decreased back and joint pain.

Note that the unpleasant joint aches experienced in a three-day fast or the first three days of a longer fast are mainly due to acid crystals, other waste products, and toxins being removed from the tissues and entering the bloodstream in large quantities. You will experience pain relief as they are eliminated from the body.

As many authors have pointed out, there is a difference between fasting and starving. Starving is going without food until death occurs. Fasting, on the other hand, is an effective way to detoxify the body by giving your body a rest for a few days.

It is my opinion, however, that we need nutrients daily, so rather than a strict water fast, I recommend a fresh enzyme-rich juice fast. In addition, some people find it easier and more enjoyable when detoxifying to follow a juice fast. In this type of fast, foods are avoided, but water and juices are consumed freely throughout the day.

Those of us who try to follow the USDA's food pyramid know that we should eat more fresh fruits and vegetables. The juice from fresh fruits and vegetables contains many natural nutrients, including vitamins, minerals, enzymes, and phytochemicals (naturally occurring plant chemicals), that can aid tremendously in the detoxification process. By drinking juice made from these fruits and vegetables, you are getting the richest, most concentrated source of their nutrients.

How to Follow a Juice Fast A juice fast is not difficult and should be followed for one to three days only and no more than once per month. Longer fasts should be supervised by a well-trained metabolic physician.

1. The day before you begin the juice fast, eat only raw fruits and vegetables. Digestive enzymes can help minimize any gastrointestinal discomfort if your body is not used to raw foods.
2. On the day of the juice fast, make and consume juices from foods that will help cleanse your body (including broccoli, carrots, apples, lettuce, cabbage, parsley, garlic, and celery), plus those fruits and vegetables high in enzymatic activity (including pineapples, papayas, kiwis, figs, garlic, and gingerroot).
3. In addition to the juice, drink a minimum of eight 8-ounce glasses of spring or distilled water per day.

4. Take a fiber supplement to augment the fiber from the fruits and vegetables when they are juiced. Powdered psyllium seed husk is almost 100 percent pure fiber bulk.
5. Take vitamin, mineral, amino acid, and enzyme supplements to augment juicing.
6. Take herbs such as cascara, buckthorn, and butternut in small doses to assist in the bowel cleanse.
7. Get as much rest as possible so that your body's energy can be geared toward healing rather than other body functions.
8. Avoid coffee and other caffeinated drinks as well as soft drinks while fasting, although herbal teas are beneficial (no sweeteners allowed).
9. Avoid tobacco in all forms.
10. Avoid any alcoholic beverages.
11. Do not exercise vigorously while fasting. Energy conservation is essential for optimal healing. Light stretching (see the exercises in chapter 9) and easy, short walks are of value. Heavy exercising overtaxes the body and interferes with body repair and detoxification.
12. Lukewarm water can be used to cleanse the skin, but extremely hot or cold water is not recommended.
13. Plenty of rest is essential while fasting. During the day, take a nap or two. Because daily activity is reduced, the body will usually require less sleep at night.
14. Enemas can be used if you become constipated, but under most situations they are unnecessary. Their use should be influenced by an individual's health status. Further, longer prefast periods (consuming only fresh vegetables and fruits) will help improve elimination. *Note:* I do believe in enemas, but if you are to use enemas as part of your colon cleanse, first consult a health care expert trained in colonic irrigations and enema therapy.
15. When you begin to break your fast, gradually return to whole, raw fruits and vegetables for the first day. Then return to your normal, healthy diet. Be sure to eat small quantities of foods frequently throughout the day. Chew foods thoroughly before swallowing.

16. As you return to whole foods, keep a record of the foods you eat and any side effects that may result. While most of us are able to handle the frequent ingestion of allergens, reintroducing an allergen after a fast may cause a headache, diarrhea, or other allergic reaction; it might even cause anaphylactic shock. It is for this reason that a physician should carefully monitor any fast longer than three days.

The following two juices are interesting ways to combine beneficial fruits and vegetables:

Vigorous Vegetable Powerhouse
- 5 carrots (without green tops)
- 1 apple, cut in small pieces (the apple helps sweeten the juice, making it more palatable)
- 4 flowerets of broccoli
- 3 leaves of lettuce
- 1–2 cabbage wedges

1. Feed the ingredients into your juicer. *Note:* Lettuce leaves may be difficult to juice alone. Therefore, you can alternate bunched-up lettuce with slices of apples or carrots, which will help push the lettuce through the juicer.
2. Drink one 8-ounce glass of this juice three times per day (upon rising, at noon, and at dinnertime).
3. Savor the flavor.

Penetrating Power Punch
- 1 bunch of parsley
- 1 cabbage wedge
- 1 clove of garlic
- 1 whole pineapple or papaya, cut in small pieces (these fruits are loaded with enzymes)
- 1 gingerroot
- 4 carrots
- 2 stalks of celery
- 1 apple, cut in small pieces

1. Feed the ingredients into your juicer.
2. Drink one 8-ounce glass of this juice three times per day (first thing in the morning or at mid-morning, at noon, and again at mid-afternoon or two hours before bed).
3. Savor the flavor.

The Importance of Water

A human can live for weeks without food but only days without water. That's because 57 percent of our total body weight is water.[1] Water plays hundreds of essential roles in the body, including regulation of body temperature. In addition, the enzymes of digestion require water to function, and circulation would be impossible without it. Water is critical in the detoxification process because it keeps the cells hydrated. In addition, without sufficient water, the kidneys and other organs would be unable to flush toxins from the body.

It is important to consume at least eight 8-ounce glasses of water every day to replace the water lost in sweat, urine, and feces as well as that lost by evaporation from the respiratory tract. Insufficient water intake can lead to dehydration, a condition particularly dangerous in infants, young children, and the elderly.

THE IMPORTANCE OF A HEALTHY DIET

In addition to calories, the food we eat provides proteins, fats, carbohydrates, vitamins, minerals, and enzymes. We need these and other nutrients to stay healthy. But consuming a diet containing sufficient nutrients also plays a positive role in the prevention and treatment of any back pain because of the role that macro- and micronutrients play in the body's metabolism. Proper nutrition gives the body fuel to function normally, to respond after injury, and to fight disease. Proper nutrition is critical for reducing stress, improving the overall health of the body, and eliminating back pain. Remember, you are what you eat. Junk foods, fried foods, and refined foods are all low in nutritional value, high in refined sugar and other simple carbohydrates, and usually high in calories. These nutrient-poor foods can put you on the fast track to back pain (as well as heart attacks and high cholesterol). They can also interfere with your recovery from back pain.

The Food Pyramid

According to the U.S. government, eating a proper diet means following the USDA's food pyramid, as illustrated in Figure 8.2. As you can see, the pyramid stresses the intake of whole cereals and grains, as well as lots of fresh fruits and vegetables, with much less emphasis on dairy foods, meats, and sweets. Unfortunately, not too many Americans follow the food pyramid. In fact, according to J. B. Cordaro, president of the Council for Responsible Nutrition, "On any given day, 40 percent of Americans do not have even one serving of fruit or fruit juice, and 20 percent have no servings of fruit or fruit juice over a period of four days."[2]

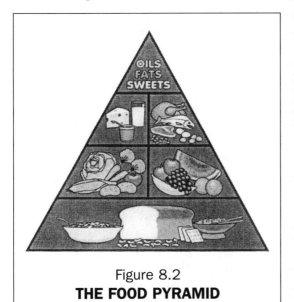

Figure 8.2
THE FOOD PYRAMID

What is the Chinese approach to proper nutrition? Taoists balance their diets with a harmony of flavors and energies. They believe that even the most wholesome foods become nutritionally useless when taken in combinations that cause fermentation and putrefaction in the gastrointestinal tract, disrupt digestion, cause conflicts in internal energy, and block nutrient absorption. This can result in toxic buildup, back and abdominal pain, and disease.

Enzymes to Jump-Start Your Life

The selection of living rather than dead foods, fresh rather than stale foods, and raw enzyme-rich or lightly cooked foods is another important concept in the Taoist diet. Live enzyme–rich foods are the key to health. Eat only foods that can rot or spoil (but be sure to eat them before they do). That is, eat live enzyme–rich foods. Remember, all (or most) enzymes are effectively killed when food is refined, radiated, pasteurized, cooked, canned, or treated with synthetic chemicals or high heat. Heat of 140°F will destroy all enzyme activity (some say 120°F or even lower).

Two groups of enzyme-rich foods are used in traditional Asian diets. One is enzyme-rich fresh raw foods, including vegetables, fruits, and grains (in Japan, they also eat raw fish). The second group consists of certain foods that have been treated with enzymes from *Aspergillus* or other microbes. These enzymes assist in the digestion of carbohydrates, fats, and proteins. Enzymatically active foods such as miso (fermented porridge from rice, soybeans, and barley), tofu (bean curd), natto (fermented soy sprouts), and other enzyme-fermented foods help spark and jump-start your day.

It is important to understand that enzymes are critical for proper digestion and metabolism of all nutrients, for overall harmony, for general body health, and for the elimination of back pain. As catalysts, enzymes affect every cell and organ in the body. Further, without proper digestion—a process in which enzymes play a key role—toxin buildup will occur and back pain can result.

Food is the fuel for your body. Therefore, give it the best fuel available. Give it premium. Plan your meals to maximize your health by following the Five-Step Jump-Start Plus Program's Dietary Do's and Don'ts.

THE FIVE-STEP JUMP-START PLUS PROGRAM DIETARY DO'S AND DON'TS

1. As much as possible, eat fresh fruits and vegetables in season. Foods not in season have been stored for months and may have been exposed to food preservatives or radiation, both of which kill active enzymes.
2. Do not eat foods sprayed with pesticides, herbicides, fungicides, or insecticides and/or foods grown close to highways.
3. Thoroughly wash and scrub all vegetables and fruits.

4. Whenever possible, eat vegetables and fruits whole, including their seeds and skins.
5. Include a lot of garlic and onions in your diet. These foods contain many beneficial phytonutrients.
6. Avoid heavy metals. Use stainless steel or glass cooking containers rather than aluminum. Also make sure that any crystal and ceramic glasses or dinnerware are free of lead.
7. Eat little or no refined sugar, refined white flour, salt, alcohol, caffeine, fat, and other potential toxin producers.
8. Proper elimination is mandatory for good health. Therefore, include adequate bulk in your diet; eat whole grains, fresh vegetables and fruits, and other complex carbohydrates. These foods have enough fiber to ensure proper elimination.
9. Drink plenty of freshly made fruit and vegetable juices (such as from pineapples, beets, and carrots).
10. Avoid excessively hot or cold foods or beverages. Extremes in temperature can overstress your body.
11. Eat frequently (five or six times) throughout the day, but eat small food portions. This gives your digestive system an opportunity to work more efficiently and does not overtax it.
12. Increase your intake of foods high in calcium (such as dairy products), B vitamins (whole grains and cereals), and vitamin C (citrus fruits), and include any other foods that are good sources of the nutrients mentioned in the discussion on supplements (see pages 109–126).
13. Eat plenty of cold-water fish, including salmon, mackerel, halibut, and herring. These fish contain omega-3 polyunsaturated fatty acids, including eicosapentaenoic acid (EPA) and decosahexanoic acid (DHA), which suppress inflammation because they suppress the synthesis of prostaglandins.

Proteins

Proteins are the body's building blocks, structural materials essential for growth and repair as well as proper cell function. Proteins are made up of about twenty common amino acids. Although the body can manufacture some amino acids (called the nonessential amino acids), there are nine of them (called the essential amino acids) that we cannot make or cannot make in adequate quantities (See Table 8.2). The essential amino acids must be obtained in the diet. Animal foods (beef, pork, and other meats; poultry; fish; milk, cheese, and eggs) are usually excellent sources of protein because they contain complete proteins (all the essential amino acids we require). Plant-derived foods can also provide protein but usually contain fewer essential amino acids.

Table 8.1

AMINO ACIDS

ESSENTIAL AMINO ACIDS	NONESSENTIAL AMINO ACIDS
Histidine	Alanine
Isoleucine	Arginine
Leucine	Asparagine
Lysine	Aspartic acid
Methionine	Cysteine
Phenylalanine	Glutamic acid
Threonine	Glutamine
Tryptophan	Glycine
Valine	Proline
	Serine
	Tyrosine

Carbohydrates

Carbohydrates provide energy to the body. This nutrient cannot be stored in significant amounts by the body. Although many Americans get their carbohydrates from sugary snacks and cola drinks, the best sources of complex carbohydrates are whole grains, fresh fruits, and fresh vegetables.

Fats

Although the current trend in food marketing is "fat free," a certain amount of fat is actually essential to health. Fats are greasy and not soluble in water. They are also the most concentrated source of food energy (they have twice as many calories per gram than do proteins or carbohydrates). Depending on their chemical structure, fats can be solid (saturated), such as those in animal foods (picture a well-marbled steak), or liquid (unsaturated), such as those in vegetables and fish.

Vitamins, Minerals, Enzymes, and Phytochemicals

Vitamins are chemical compounds that are essential in small amounts for good health and for relieving pain. Many vitamins function as coenzymes, necessary for the proper function of various enzyme systems in the body. Vitamins can be water soluble or fat soluble. The water-soluble category includes vitamin A, the B vitamins (including thiamin, riboflavin, niacin, pyridoxine, folic acid, and B_{12}), and vitamin C. Because these vitamins dissolve in water, they are not stored to any extent in the body. The fat-soluble category includes vitamins A, D, E, and K. Fat-soluble vitamins tend to be stored in the body.

Mineral elements constitute only about 4 to 5 percent of the body weight, but they are essential both as structural components and as constituents in many vital processes. Minerals include sodium, potassium, calcium, phosphorus, magnesium, and sulfur, as well as numerous trace minerals such as iron, zinc, chromium, and selenium. For some functions, it is the balance of mineral ions that is important. For example, in bone formation, the amount and ratio of calcium and phosphorus is important. For normal muscular activity, the ratio between potassium and calcium in the extracellular fluid is critical. Other minerals may act as catalysts in enzyme systems or as integral parts of organized compounds in the body, such as iron in hemoglobin, iodine in thyroxine, cobalt in vitamin B_{12}, zinc in insulin, and sulfur in thiamin and biotin.

Our food also provides vital enzymes. Enzymes are proteins naturally produced by the body that are responsible for every activity that takes place in the body. Many enzymes can be obtained in the diet in fresh, raw food. Because heat kills enzymes, it is important to eat raw fruits and vegetables as much as possible.

The use of fresh, enzyme-rich foods is an important principle in all holistic and healthy diets. Foods must be living and fresh, rather than stale or dead, and the eating of lightly cooked or raw, enzyme-rich, uncooked foods is recommended.

Unfortunately, many of today's commercially prepared "fresh" foods are radiated or chemically refined to increase their shelf life. These powerful gamma rays may kill the harmful bacteria and bugs, but the radiation also kills all the active enzymes so critical for life. The supposedly "fresh" food can sit on a shelf, without refrigeration, for weeks or months without spoiling. I have seen this and so have you.

Both Eastern and Western scientists know how fragile enzymes are and how they can be affected by such forces as high heat, radiation, moisture, synthetic chemicals, and oxygen. All of these factors are present to some degree during refining, pasteurizing, cooking, preserving, and canning of foods. Remember, all active enzymes are destroyed at temperatures of 140°F or above (and some say as low as 120°F). Most preserving methods involve heat at these, or greater, temperatures.

To illustrate how heat affects enzymes, try putting fresh, enzyme-rich pineapple in gelatin. What happens? The gelatin won't set. This is because active enzymes in the pineapple break up the protein in the gelatin and keep it from setting. However, put canned, enzyme-dead pineapple in the gelatin and the gelatin will set as pretty as a picture. This is because there are no active enzymes in the canned pineapple to break down and liquefy the gelatin. The heat of canning has effectively killed all the enzymes in the pineapple. They don't interfere with the proteins in the gelatin, so the gelatin is able to set.

A number of live, enzyme-rich foods, such as fresh fruits, vegetables, and even raw fish, are found in the traditional Asian diet. Some foods can also be treated with *Aspergillus* microbial plant enzymes, which give the food necessary enzymes for protein, fat, and carbohydrate digestion. In fact, for centuries, *Aspergillus* enzyme cultures have been used in eastern Asia for preparation of foods. Fermented foods, extremely high in enzymatic activity, include miso (fermented porridge of rice, soybean, or barley), yuba (bean-cured skin), natto (fermented soy sprouts), and tofu (bean curd).

Stir-frying is a traditional Chinese cooking method that is becoming increasingly popular throughout the world. Although temperatures are very high, stir-frying usually takes only thirty to sixty seconds. The short cooking time keeps the vital enzymes sealed inside the vegetables and meats and also keeps vital enzyme-rich juices from evaporating. Stir-fried vegetables are still a little crispy. The crispness indicates that the vegetables' internal cellular structure is still present and healthy.

If you want better nutrition than a fast-food hot dog, hamburger, or submarine sandwich can provide, try using crispy lettuce leaves instead of bread. Make a "salad in a roll." Lay out a large fresh lettuce leaf or dried and pressed sheets of seaweed (nori) on the table, then pile on raw cabbage and lettuce, fresh tomatoes, avocado, minced onions, poached asparagus, or bean sprouts. Wrap up the leaf (or leaves) and you have a delicious, wholesome meal of vital enzyme-rich foods—a great meal to revitalize the body and to fight the causes of back pain within your body.

In addition to being an important part of a nutritious diet, delicious, enzyme-rich fresh foods will allow more of your body's own enzymes to fight inflammation, disease, and the discomfort of back pain.

Phytochemicals

Food also provides phytochemicals (*phyto* means "plant"), in addition to enzymes, vitamins, minerals, proteins, nucleic acids, and other nutrients. Researchers are just beginning to investigate plant foods for their influence on human metabolism, physiology, and various common degenerative conditions. Many phytochemicals have proven disease-preventing values, including anti-inflammatory, anticancer, immune-stimulating, and cardiovascular properties. And these are nutrients found in edible vegetables and fruits! Try to increase your intake of the foods listed in Table 8.2, whose phytochemicals can help back pain.

Table 8.2

FUNCTIONAL FOOD PHYTOCHEMICALS

PHYTOCHEMICAL	PLANT SOURCE	DISEASE-FIGHTING PROPERTIES
Alpha-linolenic acid	Soy products, flaxseed, walnuts	Decreases inflammation, stimulates the immune system
Anthocyanidins	Bilberry extract (botanical cousin of the blueberry), raspberry, cranberry, red wine, grapes (skin and seeds), hawthorn, black currants, red cabbage	Maintain blood flow in small vessels, protect blood vessels, inhibit swelling, fight inflammation and free radicals
Bioflavonoids *(vitamin P) (see discussion on flavonoids, page 131)*	Pulp and rinds of most citrus fruits, quercetin, rutin	Fight inflammation, reduce capillary fragility; used to treat strains, sprains, bumps, and bruises
Curcumin	Turmeric	Used externally for wound healing
Essential fatty acids	Spirulina, seed oil, evening primrose oil and powder, black currants	Decrease inflammation, stimulate the immune system

PHYTOCHEMICAL	PLANT SOURCE	DISEASE-FIGHTING PROPERTIES
Gingerols	Ginger	Fight inflammation; potent antioxidants
Glycyrrhizins	Licorice and licorice extract	Inhibit inflammation
Lignans	Flaxseed, walnuts	Block prostaglandins involved in inflammation
Naringin *(citrus bioflavonoid)*	Rinds of grapefruits and oranges	Stabilizes membranes; antioxidant
Omega-3 fatty acids	Flaxseed, walnuts, canola oil	Reduce inflammation
Organosulfur compounds	Aged garlic extract (AGE), garlic, onions	Stimulate glutathione *s*-transferase production (a potent antioxidant), help dissolve blood clots
Polyacetylenes	Carrots, parsley, celery	Regulate prostaglandin production (prostaglandins are involved in inflammation)

(Continued)

Table 8.2 *(Continued)*

PHYTOCHEMICAL	PLANT SOURCE	DISEASE-FIGHTING PROPERTIES
Proanthocyanidins	Red grape skin extract, grape seed extract, pycnogenol, elderberry extract, hawthorn berry, bilberry, red cabbage	Potent antioxidants; strengthen blood vessel cell walls
Quercetin *(a flavonoid)*	Red wine, onions, broccoli, squash, grapes; widely distributed in the plant kingdom	Fights inflammation, reduces capillary fragility, stabilizes membranes
Rutin	Eucalyptus leaves, pagoda tree	Strengthens small capillaries (blood vessels), fights free radicals
S-allyl cysteine	Aged garlic extract	Stimulates the immune system; potent antioxidant
Salin *(or salicin)*	White willow bark extract	Decreases inflammation; relieves pain; relieves symptoms of arthritis, bursitis, and headaches
Saponins	Ginseng root, licorice, black	Fight inflammation, enhance wound

PHYTOCHEMICAL	PLANT SOURCE	DISEASE-FIGHTING PROPERTIES
	cohosh, sea cucumber, seeds of the horse chestnut, yucca	healing
Tannins	Grapes (seed and skin), red wine, green tea, oak bark, walnut hulls, and many other plants	Potent antioxidants; strengthen capillaries, relieve symptoms of rheumatism

SUPPLEMENTS

In the twelfth century, Moses Maimonides, at one time chief rabbi and physician to Saladin, sultan of Egypt and Syria, wisely said, "No illness which can be treated by diet should be treated by any other means." This is true, as far as it goes. Unfortunately, most of us don't eat a healthy diet, and few of us follow the food pyramid. Our traditional, well-balanced diets have been replaced by fast food, snack food, sweets, and TV dinners. Our Western diets are high in salt, refined sugar, red meats, and saturated fats but usually low in grains, fiber, vegetables, and fruit. These acid-forming diets of concentrated sugars, starches, and proteins cause toxification of our bodies and weaken our natural resistance to outer and inner stress, thus causing body imbalance. At the same time, they encourage the accumulation of debris from acid end products of cell decomposition, digestion, and metabolism. Whatever overtaxes our alkaline reserves also drains our potential to function. How can anyone expect to improve from a back condition when his or her body is metabolically sick? With this lifestyle, back pain seems almost inevitable.

Even those of us who try to follow the food pyramid have a difficult time, because today's growing, shipping, and processing practices grossly deplete the nutrient levels of our foods. Many of us take medications that can affect the proper digestion of foods and interfere with nutrient absorption, while others have chronic diseases that also affect nutrients in the body. Therefore, in my opinion, only by taking supplements can we ensure an optimal intake of the vitamins, minerals, enzymes, phytochemicals, and other nutrients our body requires to fight a back condition. More and more Americans are turning to supplements as an effective way to ensure optimal nutrient intake and maintain good health. In fact, it is estimated that nearly one hundred million Americans use dietary supplements.[3]

Unlike drugs, nutrients—including enzymes, minerals, and vitamins—are essential to life and bodily function. Supplements can help promote healing, reduce infection, improve joint motion, and promote nerve function. They can help decrease your level of pain and improve the strength and function of your bones, cartilage, muscles, ligaments, and tendons. Some supplements can help you sleep, while others will help your muscles to relax.

Begin by taking a good multivitamin and mineral complex, which should include antioxidants and digestive enzymes to protect, detoxify, and maintain the body. If you can't locate a supplement containing all of these nutrients, then take them separately. Then, from the following list of vitamins, minerals, enzymes, and other supplements, choose those products that can help you the most, but understand that this will vary, depending on your needs.

VIGOROUS VITAMINS

Vitamins are organic (carbon-containing) compounds that are essential in very small amounts for health, growth, and reproduction. Most vitamins must be obtained from our diet because either the body can't make them at all or it can't make them in sufficient amounts. To be healthy, we need a sufficient intake of both the fat-soluble vitamins (A, D, E, and K) and the water-soluble vitamins (B and C).

Note: It is possible to overdose on fat-soluble vitamins (vitamins A, D, E, and K). Therefore, before taking high doses of these vitamins, see a well-trained health care specialist.

Vitamin A

Vitamin A is a fat-soluble vitamin best known for its important role in maintaining normal eyesight, immune system function, and healthy skin. A deficiency of this vitamin may actually aggravate a condition and cause increased inflammation.[4] Back injuries, including sprains and strains, always involve inflammation. It's the body's way to repair any injury or infection. So a vitamin A deficiency can lead to a higher risk of disabling tissue destruction and irreversible damage. In addition, a deficiency of this vitamin is one of the major causes of blindness among children in many countries.

- Take at least 4,000 IU (international units) of vitamin A every day, in supplements or in foods (where it occurs as beta-carotene), to maintain health and ensure an adequate intake of vitamin A.

Vitamin B Complex

B complex vitamins include B_1 (thiamine), B_2 (riboflavin), B_3 (niacin), B_5 (pantothenic acid), B_6 (pyridoxine), and B_{12} (cobalamin). Most B vitamins work as coenzymes, essential for the proper function of various enzyme systems in the body. Some of the B vitamins act as "enzyme helpers" to release energy from the carbohydrates, fats, and proteins that you eat. Other B vitamins help cells to multiply. Many of these vitamins are essential to nerve health. Adequate intake of the B vitamins is important if you are to recover from back pain, regardless of its cause.

The B vitamins are all interdependent. That is, each one affects the absorption, metabolism, and excretion of the other B vitamins. For example, a folate deficiency will cause a thiamine deficiency because folate is involved in thiamine absorption. In turn, a vitamin B_{12} deficiency will keep folate from manufacturing red blood cells because B_{12} is needed to free folate.

B vitamins have been used effectively to decrease the

need for drugs, including nonsteroidal anti-inflammatory drugs (NSAIDs) such as diclofenac, often used to treat back pain. Several studies have found that combining diclofenac with B vitamins is more effective at reducing back pain than by using diclofenac alone.[5-7] These same studies have found that combining B vitamins with NSAIDs means a shorter treatment time and allows a reduction in the dosage of the NSAID. This could be very helpful in therapy, because NSAIDs are known to cause gastrointestinal irritation, headaches, dizziness, and liver damage.

Vitamin B taken alone also appears to relieve pain. M. Eckert and P. Schejbal measured the effect of a vitamin B preparation on 1,149 patients suffering from neuralgia, polyneuropathy, neuritis, and radiculopathy associated with paresthesias (abnormal burning or prickling) and pain.[8] The researchers found that treatment with the vitamin B mixture led to a clear improvement in the intensity of pain, the burning and prickling, and the muscle weakness affecting the legs. Three weeks after the first examination, the researchers again examined the study participants. They found that 69 percent of the cases had experienced a positive effect on pain because of the treatment. Muscle weakness in the legs and paresthesias improved similarly.

B vitamins may be effective on pain at the spinal level because they appear to suppress nociceptive transmission.[9] Nociceptors are pain receptors in the body that detect damage in the tissues, whether physical or chemical in nature.[10] Suppressing their transmission decreases or eliminates the sensation of pain.

In addition to reducing pain, B vitamins may also accelerate the healing process. A study reported in the *American Journal of Clinical Nutrition* found that supplemental pantothenic acid (vitamin B_5) can accelerate the normal healing process.[11] Although the exact mechanism of pantothenate's beneficial effect remains unclear, the researchers feel that it may improve the rate at which cells multiply, which would accelerate healing.

- Take at least 50 milligrams of a vitamin B complex three times every day to support neuromuscular function, feed your body's enzymes, relieve pain, and speed healing.

Vitamin C

Vitamin C is a natural antioxidant made in sufficient amounts by most animals but not by humans (nor by some primates, fish, and guinea pigs). Because our bodies don't manufacture vitamin C, we must consume it in our diet. But how many citrus fruits have you eaten today? You may need supplemental vitamin C to ensure an adequate intake of this important vitamin.

Vitamin C is essential for the proper functioning of an enzyme involved in collagen production. Collagen is the protein material from which connective tissues (such as ligaments, tendons, scars, and the foundation of bones and teeth) are made. If your back pain is due to involvement of ligaments, tendons, bony abnormalities, or any other connective tissue, you need vitamin C to ensure sufficient collagen production.

Vitamin C has been found to increase pain tolerance,[12] significantly decrease the inflammatory response, increase the rate of wound healing, and improve immune function. It benefits many common inflammatory joint conditions, including osteoarthritis.[13]

- Take at least 1,000 to 2,000 milligrams of vitamin C twice per day.
- Those who smoke, drink alcohol, or use oral contraceptives, antibiotics, or anti-inflammatory medicines require higher vitamin C intake, as do those suffering from stress and diabetes.[13]

Vitamin D

Vitamin D is a fat-soluble vitamin and an important regulator of calcium and phosphorus metabolism. It is involved in bone formation and resorption. Vitamin D is so important to bone formation that a deficiency in children will lead to rickets. Rickets is marked by restlessness, poor sleep, delayed sitting and crawling, and bowlegs (the most obvious symptom). Vitamin D also helps maintain muscle integrity, enhances calcium absorption in the intestine, and plays a role in some aspects of immune function.

Although our body can manufacture vitamin D when exposed to the sun's ultraviolet light, we may need supplemental vitamin D during the winter or whenever our exposure to the sun is minimal. Older people are at an increased risk of a vitamin D deficiency because their diets are often inadequate. Aging also brings on many physiological changes that can interfere with the absorption and utilization of this important vitamin. Drugs (including cholesterol-lowering agents) and disease can also interfere with vitamin D absorption and/or metabolism.

The consequences of a vitamin D deficiency are likely to be a reduction in bone strength and function and the development of pain.[14] Supplements may be necessary to avoid this possibility and to make sure your bones have enough of this important vitamin.

■ Take at least 500 IU daily.

Vitamin E

Vitamin E is a fat-soluble vitamin best known for its role as a potent antioxidant. Neurological changes, including peripheral neuropathy (a functional disturbance in the peripheral nervous system), posterior column dysfunction (a dysfunction in one of the columns of the spinal cord), and cerebellar ataxia (failure of muscular coordination and irregularity of muscular action), can occur because of vitamin E deficiency.[15]

Vitamin E appears to have analgesic activity. That is, it can help relieve pain. In an English study, forty-two patients suffering from rheumatoid arthritis were given 600 milligrams of vitamin E (alpha-tocopherol) twice per day.[16] After twelve weeks, pain in the morning, evening, and after a chosen activity was significantly decreased.

Another study observed the effect of vitamin E on the degenerative process occurring in humans with spondylosis.[17] Spondylosis is an ankylosis, or immobility, of a vertebral joint, often caused by arthritis. The researchers discovered that most of the patients had lower than normal serum vitamin E levels. Administration of 100 milligrams of vitamin E daily for a three-week period resulted in complete pain relief, plus a significant increase in serum vitamin E levels. The findings strongly indicate that "vitamin E is effective in curing spondylosis and most probably due to its antioxidant activity."[17]

■ Take at least 400 IU of vitamin E daily to fight free radicals and ensure an adequate intake.

Vitamin K

Vitamin K is a fat-soluble vitamin that activates blood-clotting proteins, proteins in bone and kidney, and the formation of other proteins that contain gamma-carboxyglutamic acid (GLA). Its main function is the coagulation of blood. Because vitamin K is synthesized by intestinal bacteria, deficiencies generally occur only in infants whose intestinal flora has not yet been established, in children and adults receiving antibiotic or anticoagulant therapy, and in individuals with disease conditions that interfere with intestinal absorption.

Evidence suggests that at least half of the vitamin K required by humans is normally synthesized by bacteria in the intestine. In rare cases, vitamin K deficiency may occur with fat malabsorption, which is common in alcoholics.

■ Take at least 50 micrograms of vitamin K daily to ensure an adequate intake.

MIGHTY MINERALS

Minerals are inorganic substances (neither animal nor vegetable) that are responsible for a number of activities within the body. Some minerals function as cofactors, important components of various enzyme systems in the body. Others are important for strong bones and teeth because they provide skeletal strength and rigidity. Some regulate the balance of electrolytes and fluids, while still others regulate nerve transmission and muscle function.

Some minerals, including calcium, chloride, magnesium,

phosphorus, potassium, and sodium, are required in amounts ranging from several hundred milligrams to one or more grams a day. Others, including boron, chromium, cobalt, copper, iodine, iron, manganese, selenium, and zinc, are required in much smaller amounts. Several of these minerals can be of tremendous help in the treatment of back pain.

Minerals are found in most foods but usually only in limited amounts. If you eat a low-calorie diet for a long period of time, you run the risk of developing mineral deficiencies. Deficiencies can also develop if you're taking medication that interferes with the absorption and metabolism of minerals. For instance, antacids, taken by millions of Americans every day, increase the demand for calcium, iron, and phosphorus. Diuretics increase the demand for potassium, calcium, magnesium, and zinc (as well as a number of important vitamins). Further, alcoholism, renal disease, or gastrointestinal diseases can also cause deficiencies because they alter the way the body breaks down, absorbs, and metabolizes minerals.

Boron

The trace mineral boron appears to be an important nutrient for healthy bones and joints, although an absolute requirement for boron has not yet been definitely established for humans. Researchers have learned, however, that boron supplementation is effective in wound healing and in fighting osteoporosis and inflammation.

Boron appears to be an effective and safe treatment for some forms of arthritis,[18] and other conditions that involve inflammation.[19] Findings indicate that people with arthritis have lower boron concentrations in bones, femur heads (the femur is the bone that runs from the pelvis to the knee), and synovial fluid than those who don't suffer from arthritis. One study found that 50 percent of osteoarthritis patients taking 6 milligrams of boron per day experienced improvement of symptoms, compared to only 10 percent of those receiving a placebo.[18]

■ Take 6 milligrams of boron per day for better joints, to fight inflammation, and to improve calcium uptake.

Calcium

Calcium is used by the body for building bones and teeth and for maintaining bone strength. In fact, most of the body's calcium, perhaps as much as 99 percent, is held in the bones and teeth.[20] The remainder of the body's calcium circulates in the bloodstream. Calcium also plays important roles in muscle contraction, nerve transmission, blood clotting, and maintenance of cell membranes.[20] Calcium aids in the functioning of several enzymes in the body and also regulates the secretion of various hormones.

■ Take 2,000 milligrams of calcium every day for strong teeth and bones, proper muscle contraction, and proper nerve transmission.

Magnesium

Magnesium is used in building bones, maintaining glucose metabolism, manufacturing proteins, releasing energy from muscle storage, and regulating body temperature. It is involved in muscle contraction and blood clotting and plays a role in the conduction of nerve impulses to the muscles.

Magnesium is so important to nerve and muscle health that symptoms of a deficiency can include muscular twitching and tremors, muscle weakness, and leg and foot cramps. A deficiency can also cause shaky hands, insomnia, and an irregular heartbeat.[21]

■ Take at least 1,000 milligrams of magnesium every day.

Manganese

Manganese plays an important role in the normal functioning of the central nervous system. It is also a part of enzymes that prevent lipid peroxidation by free radicals and also those enzymes that assist in urea synthesis.

The symptoms of manganese deficiency include bone abnormalities (such as swollen and enlarged joints, shortened and thickened limbs, and curvature of the spine), growth defects, disturbances in lipid and carbohydrate metabolism, reproductive dysfunction, and central nervous system manifestations. It has also been suggested that a manganese deficiency can be a potential underlying factor in the development of hip abnormalities, joint disease, congenital malformations, and osteoporosis.[22]

■ Take at least 5 milligrams of manganese every day for better joints and a properly functioning central nervous system.

Potassium

Potassium assists in muscle contraction and is important in sending nerve impulses. It promotes normal growth, maintains proper water balance between body fluids and cells, and is necessary for cellular enzymes to work properly. Symptoms of a potassium deficiency can include muscular weakness, abnormal heart rhythm, lethargy, and impaired nerve impulses and muscle contraction. When muscle contractions occur in the back or legs, they can result in muscle imbalance and back pain.

■ Take at least 100 milligrams of potassium every day.

Selenium

Selenium works with vitamin E as an antioxidant and is part of the antioxidant enzyme glutathione peroxidase. Low selenium intake results in poor nutritional status as well as low tissue levels of glutathione peroxidase and can lead to severe chronic disorders such as cardiovascular diseases and cancer.

■ Take at least 200 micrograms of selenium every day.

Silicon

The ultratrace element silicon (silica) is essential for proper growth and development and collagen formation. It has a wide spectrum of applications, including bolstering connective tissue matrix and enhancing bone formation and calcium uptake. Silicon contributes to the resilience and architecture of connective tissue because it functions as a biological cross-linking agent. It helps fight osteoporosis and atherosclerosis.

■ Take at least 25 milligrams of silicon every day for strong bones, healthy connective tissue, and improved calcium absorption and utilization.

Zinc

Zinc is one of the most essential trace minerals found in our bodies. It is in every tissue and tissue fluid. Of all the trace minerals, only iron is found in greater concentrations. Zinc is especially beneficial in the treatment of back pain because it is required for general growth and maintenance of all tissues and assists in wound healing. It plays a part in blood formation, affects thyroid hormone function, interacts with platelets in blood clotting, is needed to produce retinal (the active form of vitamin A) in visual pigments, affects learning and behavior, is essential to normal salt-taste perception, helps protect the body from heavy metal poisoning, and is essential in the production of sperm and in fetal development. In addition, zinc is a component of hundreds of enzymes and thus is involved in most metabolic processes.

■ Take at least 50 milligrams of zinc per day to stay healthy.

THE STRAIGHT SCOOP ON ENZYMES

Many people ask me if enzyme supplements can help relieve back and joint pain. My response is an emphatic yes! And they do so in many ways. Enzymes can help you live a longer, healthier life, pain-free.

Enzymes are necessary for almost every activity in the body. In fact, no action can take place in the body without enzymatic activity. Without enzymes, life cannot exist. Enzymes keep us tuned up. They function as catalysts, accelerating a reaction or causing a reaction to take place. They make digestion possible, help regulate our metabolism, and keep us performing at top speed. Enzymes occur naturally in all living things—microbes, animals, plants, and humans. If it's alive, it has enzymes.

However, aging, illness, or injury can cause our body's production of enzymes to decrease, and the enzymes produced may have a lower activity level.

Enzyme Supplements

In the United States, enzyme supplements have primarily been used to improve digestion, but they are also extremely effective at fighting inflammation and back pain. Consider the case of a soccer coach who injured his back after demonstrating a soccer kick. He immediately felt a sharp, stabbing pain in his lower back that radiated down into the right leg (the pain was especially severe in the calf). He began taking enzyme supplements shortly after his injury.

According to the orthopedic surgeon who evaluated the coach some nine weeks after the injury, there was little doubt that this man had suffered an injury to a lumbar disk with right leg nerve pain. The orthopedist felt that the coach had made a remarkably good recovery and noted that he was essentially symptom free at the time of examination. The doctor was amazed at his swift recovery and concluded that the patient required no further medical treatment.

Enzymes are especially effective at treating the inflammation that results from injury. By breaking up the debris in the injured area and allowing blood vessels to "unclog," enzymes effectively decrease pain and swelling and can lead to a more rapid repair of the injured area. Bromelain, papain, pancreatin (which contains many enzymes, including trypsin and chymotrypsin), serratiopeptidase, and other enzyme combinations are often used to fight inflammation.

An abundance of research shows that in addition to reducing back pain, enzymes can also improve digestive problems, injuries, arthritis, cancer, gynecological problems, fibrocytis, circulatory problems, viruses (including AIDS), and multiple sclerosis. They can improve immune function (and break up antigen-antibody complexes), detoxify the body, improve nutrient absorption, and slow the aging process. I cover this in depth in my books *Enzymes and Enzyme Therapy: How To Jump Start Your Way to Lifelong Good Health* (Los Angeles: Keats Publishing, 1994) and *The Complete Book of Enzyme Therapy* (Garden City Park, N.Y.: Avery Publishing, 1999).

ENZYMES AT A GLANCE

- An enzyme deficiency can be the difference between health and disease.
- The majority of enzyme names end in *ase* and are named for the substance (called the substrate) they act upon. For instance, the enzyme lipase works on lipids (fats), while protease works on protein.

ENZYME EFFECTIVENESS IS INFLUENCED BY:

- Acid (low-pH) or base (high-pH) environments.
- Temperature. Enzymes are destroyed under certain conditions of heat.
- Substrates. Enzymes are very specific, and each enzyme only works with certain fats, carbohydrates, proteins, or other substrates.
- Coenzymes (vitamins) and cofactors (minerals). Coenzymes and cofactors are needed for certain enzymes to do their jobs. Vitamin C and the B vitamins are coenzymes, while minerals such as zinc, copper, and iron are cofactors.
- Enzyme inhibitors.

ENZYMES WORK TO FIGHT BACK PAIN BY:

- Decreasing swelling, pain, and inflammation without suppressing immune system activity (as do cortisone products)
- Restoring local and overall blood circulation
- Increasing the speed of healing
- Inhibiting the formation and stimulating the breakup, of small blood clots
- Permitting healing agents normally found in the blood to reach the injured area and permitting waste products to be removed more quickly

THE FOLLOWING ANTIOXIDANT ENZYMES HELP TO FIGHT FREE RADICALS:

- Glutathione peroxidase (requires selenium)
- Superoxide dismutase (requires zinc and copper)
- Catalase

SOURCES OF ENZYME SUPPLEMENTS INCLUDE:
- Plants (mainly pineapples, papayas, and figs)
- Microbes, such as fungi and bacteria (these are often called "plant-derived" enzymes)
- Animals (including cattle and pigs)

METHODS OF ADMINISTRATION INCLUDE:
- Orally, in lozenges (dissolved in the mouth) or oral tablets (designed either to break down in the stomach or to pass through intact). These supplements are widely available at health food, drug, or grocery stores. Some oral enzyme supplements are coated to prevent their breakdown in the stomach and allow for their release in the small intestine.

- Topically, certain enzymes are available as ointments that can be spread over the involved area.
- By injection. Injectable enzymes are available from a physician and are usually administered in a hospital setting.

The Four Ways That Supplemental Enzymes Can Help Back Pain

With back and joint pain and conditions that cause back pain, supplemental enzymes have a multiple purpose:

1. Enzyme supplements that are designed to be absorbed from the gut into the body's bloodstream and act directly on specific organs and cells within the body are called *systemic enzymes*. Systemic enzyme therapy can decrease the effects of inflammation, improve circulation, stimulate immune function, fight free radicals, and fight enemy viruses and bacteria. Systemic enzymes should be taken between meals to be most effective.

2. Proper digestion is important to maintain a normal supply of nutrients to the musculoskeletal system so as to maintain a healthy, pain-free back and joints and help

fight inflammation and disease. Enzymes are critical for proper digestion of food and nutrients. Digestive enzyme supplements break down a broad range of protein-, fat-, and carbohydrate-containing foods and ensure normal elimination of toxic waste products. Proteases break up proteins, amylases break up carbohydrates, and lipases break up fats. Digestive enzymes replace the enzymes destroyed by cooking, chemicals, and radiation of foods. Digestive enzymes should be taken just before or with meals for best effect.

3. EASE™ stands for Enzyme Absorption Systems Enhancers. EASE supplements are combinations of enzymes and other nutrients used to treat specific conditions. With EASE products, absorption and bioavailability of food extracts, herbs, and other nutrients are improved. For example, thirty-five years of scientific research have shown the enzyme bromelain to improve the effectiveness of antibiotics.[23–27]

4. Enzymes aid in overall health, wellness, and prevention of illness. Enzymes are a natural, essential component of all fresh, raw foods and are necessary to activate and catalyze other nutrients in those foods. Although this could be considered a subdivision of the EASE category (first discussed in my book *The Complete Book of Enzyme Therapy* [Garden City Park, N.Y.: Avery Publishing Group, 1999]), it also has its own specific place in health care.

WHAT'S AVAILABLE IN ENZYME SUPPLEMENTS?

The enzyme supplements of most benefit in the treatment of inflammation (and therefore back conditions) are primarily proteolytic enzymes. This group includes bromelain, pancreatin, papain, trypsin, chymotrypsin, and microbial proteases.

The proper dosage will vary, depending on your health status, age, and the severity of your injury or illness. A good rule of thumb is to follow the label directions. However, generally speaking, acute injuries and inflammation require higher initial doses, sometimes two to three or more times the base dose. Acute injuries usually show some change within a few days to a few weeks, but chronic conditions may take longer. You may not see a change for some four weeks with certain conditions (such as rheumatoid arthritis), but be patient. It takes time. When you are pain free, you may return to a maintenance dose for general health as per the label's directions. Remember, because you are dealing with inflammation and back pain, you should take the enzymes between meals— that is, at least an hour after meals or an hour before meals. Otherwise, the enzymes will be used by the body to digest the meal rather than fight inflammation.

Bromelain

Bromelain is an enzyme taken from the stem of the unripened pineapple. Throughout history, many tribes from around the world have used pineapple for its potent anti-inflammatory activity. Bromelain is especially helpful in back conditions (including those involving sprains, strains, sore muscles, bruises, and surgery) because of its ability to inhibit inflammation.

As mentioned earlier, inflammation involves prostaglandins. Typically, the symptoms of inflammation will subside in less than five days when bromelain is used.

- Bromelain is a *selective prostaglandin inhibitor.* It favors those compounds that fight inflammation and decreases the formation of the "bad" prostaglandins. Bromelain does not affect the "good" prostaglandins that promote the healing process.
- By inhibiting the "bad" prostaglandins, bromelain decreases swelling and pain (segments of the inflammatory reaction) and allows the body's own immune system to return to normal.
- Bromelain encourages fibrinolysis (the breakup of fibrin). Our body produces fibrin to seal wounds, among other things. By encouraging the breakup of fibrin, bromelain can help decrease swelling and inflammation.
- A high dose of bromelain, 750 to 1,500 milligrams per day, is needed to obtain meaningful results.
- Bromelain activity is calculated mainly in GDUs (gelatin

dissolving units) or MCUs (milk clotting units). Aim for an activity level of approximately 1,200 GDU or better. One GDU is equal to 1.5 MCU.

■ Bromelain also is effective as a digestive aid: it breaks down some antigen-antibody complexes (a major cause of tissue destruction in autoimmune diseases) and can fight a number of conditions, including cancer.

Pancreatin

Pancreatin is an enzyme usually taken from fresh hog or bovine pancreas, which contains a number of different enzymes including amylases, lipases, and proteases (such as trypsin and chymotrypsin).

■ Pancreatin is used to fight inflammation and back pain, to improve digestion, and to effectively treat pancreatic insufficiency.

■ Vegetarians may use papain and bromelain (protein-digesting enzymes from papaya and pineapple, respectively) as substitutes for pancreatin.

■ The proper dose of pancreatin is based on the product's activity level. Pancreatin's activity is rated against a standard established by the United States Pharmaceopoeia (USP). Each "X" of a pancreatin product's activity contains not less than 25 USP units of amylase activity, not less than 2 USP units of lipase activity, and not less than 25 USP units of protease activity. A higher strength or potency of pancreatin is found in multiples of "X." For example, a designation of 10X USP would indicate that a product is ten times stronger than government USP standards. Higher-strength pancreatin products are preferred to lower-potency products.

■ For back pain, take 750 to 1,500 milligrams of pancreatin three times per day between meals.

Papain

Papain is a proteolytic enzyme taken from the milky juice (latex) of the unripened fruit of the tropical papaya (*Carica papaya*). Because of its proteolytic activity, papain has received superior ratings for its ability to reduce swelling and decrease recovery time after traumatic sports and other injuries.

- Papain effectively treats inflammation and swelling, accelerates wound healing, and helps prevent scar tissue malformation.
- Papain is especially effective as a digestive aid, improving the digestion of protein. There is some evidence that it is also effective in treating a malabsorption syndrome that results because of gluten intolerance.
- Papain breaks down antigen-antibody complexes in immune reactions.
- For back pain, take at least four 800-milligram papain tablets three times a day between meals.

Serratiopeptidase

Serratiopeptidase is a proteolytic enzyme made from microbial sources. It appears to be very effective at fighting inflammation.

- Serratiopeptidase reduces swelling (edema).
- Serratiopeptidase stimulates the immune system.
- Serratiopeptidase improves the efficacy of antibiotics.
- Serratiopeptidase is effective at treating a number of inflammatory conditions including arthritis, carpal tunnel syndrome, and sprains and strains.

Other Helpful Enzymes

Other helpful enzymes include microbial proteases, trypsin, and chymotrypsin. These and other proteolytic enzymes can help reduce inflammation, swelling, and pain. Also of benefit are lipases (enzymes that break up lipids and fats) and amylases (enzymes that break up carbohydrates). Not only are these enzymes effective in improving digestion, they are often included in enzyme combinations to work synergistically and improve the enzymes' activity.

PROOF OF PAIN RELIEF

Just imagine what it would be like if you had no back pain—if you could bend over, twist, or turn without discomfort. Theoretically and practically, proteolytic enzymes can help you achieve that goal.

Numerous studies show fast relief from pain, swelling, and inflammation with proteolytic enzymes.[28–32] In one study with the enzyme trypsin, 94.3 percent of 538 patients experienced dramatic and rapid reduction of pain.[32] In another study, 87 out of 100 professional and amateur athletes using papaya found marked improvement in their injuries, especially a decrease in pain and swelling as well as a return to full, pain-free mobility.[30] Policemen and firemen used bromelain to prevent and treat inflammation, swelling, and pain in various injuries such as strains, sprains, and fractures.[31] Of those studied, 62.5 percent healed faster than those not taking enzymes. In a study of football players over two consecutive seasons, there was a 31 percent decrease in time lost from playing for 28 professional football players taking trypsin and chymotrypsin.[32]

In a very interesting study, J. P. Tarayre and H. Lauressergues studied the effects of proteolytic enzymes in combination with bioflavonoids and ascorbic acid and compared them with the effects obtained from common nonsteroidal anti-inflammatory substances, such as flufenamic acid, aspirin, phenylbutazone (Butazoladin), and indomethacin.[33] The regime was used to prevent and treat a number of different conditions, including dextran-induced swelling, histamine-caused wheals, and carrageenan-caused swelling. A more significant decrease in inflammation occurred with the use of a nutritional approach in contrast to treatment with classic pharmacological drugs. Anti-inflammatories had a minor effect on the carrageenan-caused swelling, while proteolytic enzymes had a positive effect in reducing inflammation. The dextran-induced swelling was completely nonresponsive to the classic anti-inflammatories.

In my study conducted at Portland State University with Leo Marty, director of sports medicine, we found that football players taking enzymes improved and experienced reductions in swelling, pain, and inflammation twice as fast as those not taking enzymes.[34] They also returned to play football twice as fast.

WHY WE NEED MORE ENZYMES AS WE AGE

As we age, our body's ability to produce enzymes decreases, and the enzymes produced are not as active. Therefore, the body's proteolytic enzymes are not as effective. This is one of the main reasons for increased back pain (and pain in general), decreased rate of healing, tissue breakdown, nutrient malabsorption, and increased chronic diseases such as back conditions, cancer, and cardiovascular disorders.

By taking increased enzyme supplementation, we can continue to give the body the nutrients it requires.

What's in the Stores?

Enzyme supplements are essential in today's fast-paced, stress-filled, enzyme-dead fast-food society. Enzyme supplements are essential for digestion and detoxification, and for fighting any number of conditions, including inflammation, sports injuries, autoimmune conditions, viral infections, skin problems, cardiovascular disorders, and cancer.

There are many fine enzyme manufacturers. However, there are some that I would specifically like to mention that produce enzymes and enzyme combinations (enzyme combinations are formulated to work together synergistically).

Wobenzym N is produced by Naturally Vitamins and includes a combination of bromelain, papain, pancreatin, trypsin, chymotrypsin, and the bioflavonoid rutin. These enzymes can be taken as digestive aids (taken before meals), or as systemic enzymes (if taken between meals).

Infla-Zyme Forte, produced by American Biologics, is a combination of antioxidants and enzymes used for digestion and to fight inflammation and serious chronic conditions such as atheroslerosis, AIDS autoimmune diseases, and cancer. Infla-Zyme Forte contains bromelain, papain, chymotrypsin,

ENZYMES IN THE FIGHT AGAINST BACK PAIN

- Enzymes can fight back pain because they inhibit inflammation, restore circulation, speed healing, and break up blood clots.
- An ounce of prevention is worth a pound of cure. Enzymes taken before you perform physically demanding activity can help speed healing should an injury occur.
- To fight the back pain, take enzymes on an empty stomach at least one to one and a half hours before or after a meal, with water or juice. As a digestive aid, take enzymes from thirty minutes to just before or with meals.
- In cases of acute injuries, begin taking enzymes as soon as possible.
- As pain and swelling decrease, take a daily maintenance dose (follow label directions).
- The benefits of enzyme therapy parallel those of other therapies, such as corticosteroids, NSAIDs, or gold (often used in treating rheumatoid arthritis) but without the potentially serious and long-term side effects of those drugs.

For further information on enzymes, please see my books on enzymes: *Enzymes and Enzyme Therapy: How to Jump Start Your Way to Lifelong Good Health* (Keats Publishing, 1994), *The Complete Book of Enzyme Therapy* (Avery Publishing Group, 1999), *Enzymes: Nature's Energizers* (Keats Publishing, 1997), and *Bromelain: The Active Enzyme That Helps Us Make the Most of What We Eat* (Keats Publishing, 1998).

trypsin, pancreatin, amylase, lipase, the antioxidant enzymes catalase, superoxide dismutase plus zinc, the bioflavonoid rutin, and L-cystine. Depending on the severity of the condition, dosage can range from two to three tablets between meals to six or even ten tablets three times per day.

Mega Zyme by Enzymatic Therapy is a multi-enzyme product that contains pancreatic enzymes, trypsin, papain, bromelain, amylase, lipase, lysozyme, and chymotrypsin. It has the highest potency (10X) pancreatic enzyme available to help break down proteins, fats, and carbohydrates in the gastrointestinal tract.

In addition, a number of other companies worth mentioning include Amano Enzymes, National Enzyme Company, Sabinsa, Prevail, and Physiologics. These companies provide plant and microbial enzymes. Their enzymes include amylase, lipase, protease, cellulase, sucrase, maltase, and lactase.

OTHER SUPPLEMENTAL HELPERS
Adrenal Glandulars
The human body contains a number of glands that produce hormones. For instance, the pancreas produces insulin, while the pituitary produces growth hormone. Of special interest to back pain sufferers are the adrenal glands, which produce epinephrine, norepinephrine, and corticosteroids (best known because of their role in controlling inflammation). In fact, many people take prescription forms of corticosteroids to fight inflammation and the pain it creates.

Animals have glands that function in many of the same ways as human glands. In fact, many people believe that taking an extract made from an animal gland can help to improve the function of the corresponding gland in the human body. Adrenal glandulars are a good example. Usually extracted from the adrenal glands of cattle, supplements made from this extract have been used to fight inflammation, stress, and adrenal exhaustion. It is for these reasons that adrenal glandulars might be of benefit to those suffering from back pain.

Manufacturers produce any number of adrenal glandulars of varying strengths. For best results, follow the directions on the label.

Aged Garlic Extract
Aged garlic extract (AGE) is an extract made from garlic and aged under controlled conditions. Over the last few years, researchers have focused on the benefits of sulfur-containing compounds in garlic. These water-soluble com-

pounds (such as *s*-allyl cysteine, or SAC) are odorless, stable, and safe. Precisely because they are water soluble, your chance of overdosing is greatly reduced. In addition, the AGE form of garlic seems to be absorbed more easily than oil-soluble forms. Aged garlic extract and SAC help fight inflammation, free radicals, cardiovascular disorders, and cancer and can lower cholesterol, boost immune function, combat stress, and improve memory.[35–39] Furthermore, AGE has been shown to fight both chemical and physical stress and fatigue.[40–42]

Because there are many forms of AGE on the market, for the best results follow the dosage recommendations on the label.

Amino Acid Complex

Amino acids are the structural units of all proteins, the "building blocks" of the entire body. They form enzymes, peptides, antibodies, and hormones, and they help the body maintain a correct acid-base balance and a proper fluid balance.

A deficiency of any of the amino acids can interfere with proper body function. Fortunately, supplemental amino acids can help replace any missing amino acids and may also help reduce pain levels.

For instance, carnitine is a naturally occurring amino acid found in the liver and in skeletal muscle.[43] A recent study by M. A. Giamberardino and colleagues found that taking 3 grams of carnitine per day for three weeks significantly decreased tenderness and pain in subjects performing twenty minutes of extreme effort of the quadriceps.[44] Excessive muscular effort can cause muscle damage and delayed muscle soreness, which do not respond to common medical treatment using analgesic agents. This can have a negative effect on back pain relief. The researchers found that carnitine administration resulted in a protective effect against damage and pain caused by extreme muscle effort.

For best results, take a good amino acid complex. To ensure adequate intake and because supplements vary in strength and content by manufacturer, follow the directions on the label.

Bioflavonoids

Bioflavonoids (part of the flavonoid group) are naturally occurring compounds widely distributed in the plant kingdom, especially in fruits (such as citrus fruits) and vegetables.

Bioflavonoids and other flavonoids are probably best known for their ability to improve capillary strength. Capillaries are very small blood vessels that spread throughout the body, like the threads of an intricate lace tablecloth. These small vessels supply nutrients to, and remove wastes from, every cell. Capillaries can be weakened or damaged when you are injured. When this occurs, nutrients around the area can't get in and waste products can't get out. This can contribute to the signs of inflammation, such as redness, swelling, heat, and pain. Flavonoids are especially effective in treating strains, sprains, bruises, and other injuries because of their effect on inflammation. Quercetin and rutin are two well-known flavonoids frequently used for this purpose. Flavonoids are also potent antioxidants and support vitamin C by increasing its absorption and preserving its action.

To keep your capillaries strong and thereby improve circulation to healing tissues, take 350 milligrams of bioflavonoids three times per day.

Boswellic Acids (Boswellin)

Nowhere is the role of prolonged anti-inflammatory treatment more important than in chronic inflammatory conditions, best exemplified by the various forms of arthritis and back pain. And nowhere is the safety factor of prolonged treatment more paramount than in the treatment of arthritis. The fact is, however, that most of the NSAIDs cause gastrointestinal irritation, which seriously limits their long-term use.

The boswellic acids or acids derived from *Boswellia serrata* (also known as frankincense) tree resin are considered a form of safe and effective anti-inflammatory nutraceutical. In one experiment, boswellic acids were compared with a common anti-inflammatory drug, phenylbutazone, and unlike phenylbutazone, boswellic acids did not produce the gastric ulceration in experimental animals.

Capsaicin

Capsaicin is a nutraceutical ingredient contained in an extract from *Capsicum annum* fruits (cayenne pepper), which is recognized by the FDA for topical application in pain-relieving preparations. Capsaicin is a compound responsible for the pungent taste of cayenne pepper. Capsaicin works in very low concentrations (0.025 percent) by whipping away the pain-sensation-causing chemicals from the nerve endings.

Curcuminoids

The term *curcuminoids* applies to three nutraceuticals derived from the roots of turmeric (*Curcuma longa*). These are brilliantly yellow phenolic principals that have a broad antioxidant action termed bioprotectant as well as the anti-inflammatory action comparable to that of NSAIDs. Turmeric is listed by the FDA as an herb generally recognized as safe. Due to their safety and efficacy, curcuminoids may be regarded as a logical choice for an anti-inflammatory composition, particularly with boswellic acids and glucosamine, when a prolonged treatment of the condition is required.

Glucosamine

Glycosaminoglycans in the body form a ground substance or a tissue glue, which is the most important element of the connective (gluing) tissue. Thus the wasting away or "chipping away" of the glycosaminoglycans, as in the inflammatory process of arthritis, leads to continuously worsening joint disfigurement and limited mobility. Supplementing glucosamine means supporting the pool of glycosaminoglycans and replenishing what was taken away by the inflammation.

Glucosamine Sulfate

Glucosamine is an amino sugar produced in the body and necessary for connective tissue formation. Glucosamine helps to maintain and generate the elasticity and thickness of synovial fluid in the joints between the vertebrae. Tissues in the joints become damaged when the lubricating synovial fluid becomes watery and thin. Cartilage and bones painfully scrape against each other if the protective cushioning is lost. Severe pain and nerve injury can occur when this happens in the spine.

Since glucosamine is a small, naturally occurring molecule, nearly 90 percent is absorbed when ingested orally, according to human and animal studies.[45,46] Of added importance is that 30 percent of an oral dose is kept by the musculoskeletal system for extended periods of time.[47] Glucosamine is not toxic.

Glucosamine is available in two forms: glucosamine sulfate and glucosamine hydrochloride. Both forms are similar, but some sources indicate that the sulfate form requires higher doses in order to obtain the same results as the hydrochloride form.

Therefore, for better joints, and to nourish cartilage, ligaments, and tendons, take 1,500 to 2,000 milligrams of glucosamine sulfate every day with meals. Glucosamine sulfate is often combined with chondroitin sulfate in supplement form.

Green Barley Extract

Green barley extract contains a compound commonly called 2-0-GIV (2'-0-glycosylisovitexin), reported to be stronger than vitamin C or E as an antioxidant and free radical fighter.[48,49] Free radicals and the cross-linking they promote can be of concern in soft tissue injuries and back pain in particular. In addition, 2-0-GIV reduces inflammation,[50] stimulates the immune system, lowers cholesterol, and fights cancer and cardiovascular disease.[48,49]

Green barley extract can be taken anytime during the day. Many people take it for an energy boost in addition to its other health qualities. For best results, follow label directions.

Methylsulfonylmethane (MSM)

Methylsulfonylmethane (MSM) is a form of sulfur derived from the ocean. MSM has been used as a dietary supplement for many years. MSM improves the elasticity of the tissue and encourages tissue repair. Tests indicate that MSM can accelerate wound-healing and may be effective at treating pain. MSM treats the cause of inflammation, helping to restore the normal flow of fluids through the tissues. For pain relief and to fight inflammation, take at least 2,000 milligrams of MSM daily. MSM seems to be more effective when taken in conjunction with vitamin C.

Combination Treatments

As much as the glucosamine replacement is a step in the right direction, it is not sufficient to provide what is continuously taken away, but rather an additional treatment is appropriate that would effectively reduce or prevent the "chipping away" of glycosaminoglycans. Such a treatment is provided by combining glucosamine supplementation with anti-inflammatory boswellic acids and curcuminoids. Although the mechanisms of boswellic acids, curcuminoids, and glucosamine are different, they support each other's action, and combined may afford more efficient management of arthritis, joint, and back pain.

HERBS FOR HEALTH

For centuries, herbs were one of the main medicines available for human use. Through trial and error, early humans found that some plants could speed wound healing, others could relieve a headache, while still others could relax and calm an injured warrior.

Many of today's medicines have their basis in old-time herbal cures. For instance, white willow contains salicin, a natural precursor to aspirin. Some herbs serve as potent pain relievers. Other herbs can help fight the inflammation that so often accompanies and may even be the cause of back pain. Several herbs improve circulation, helping the bloodstream to carry nutrients and oxygen to the damaged site, while still other herbs can help you relax, improve your sleep habits, or improve immune function when associated with back pain.

What Part of the Herb Is Used to Heal?

Herbs are a wondrous gift from nature. Every part of a plant may have medicinal value. That includes the twigs, leaves, flowers, seeds, and roots. In some plants, such as the gingerroot, even the underground fleshy stems (called *rhizomes*) can send out shoots, forming new plants.

Herbs have a variety of application techniques:

- *Compresses.* Herbal compresses are made by soaking cloth in a cold or warm herbal solution and then placing the cloth directly on the area of injury.
- *Decoctions (or tea).* Decoctions are made from the root, bark, berry, leaves, or seed of a plant. Unless your herbalist or physician directs otherwise, simmer (do not boil) the herb for about twenty to thirty minutes.
- *Essential oils.* These are oils extracted from herbs or other vegetation by cold pressing or steam distillation. Essential oils should not be taken internally.
- *Extracts.* Herbal extracts are concentrated herbal preparations formed by pressing the herbs and then soaking them in water or alcohol.
- *Infusions.* To make an infusion, steep (do not boil) the flowers, leaves, or other delicate plant parts for up to ten minutes in hot water.
- *Ointments.* Powdered or pressed herbs, tea, or extracts are mixed with a salve, then applied to the affected tissue.
- *Poultices.* Poultices are moist, hot concentrations of herbs spread over loose cloth such as muslin and applied to the affected area. Poultices are useful with inflammations.
- *Powder.* Herbs ground to a powder can be placed in tablets or capsules.
- *Syrup.* Syrup is formed when herbs are added to a sugar solution and boiled until thick.
- *Salves.* A salve is a thick ointment made with the addition of herbs. Salves are effective in treating inflammation, sores, and bruises.
- *Tinctures.* Herbal tinctures are solutions prepared with herbs and alcohol.
- *Vinegars.* Herbs can be placed in various vinegars derived from rice, malt, or raw apple cider. Allow to stand two weeks or so before using.

The following herbs are especially beneficial in the treatment of back pain. Some of them have a long history of use in Europe and the Americas, while others are known primarily in the East. Herbs are very popular in China. In fact, more than fifteen hundred different herbs are used by some 50 percent of the people in China.[51] In addition, over a thousand herbal remedies have been patented in China, and many are exported to other countries. In the United States, traditional Chinese herbs are becoming increasingly popular. *Note:* In the following list, we note the herb's botanical name and, where possible, its Chinese name.

- Achyranthes (botanical name, *Achyranthes bidentata*; in Chinese, niu xi or niu hsi). The root of the achyranthes, used for centuries in Chinese medicine, is effective as a diuretic; it also promotes circulation and functions as a kidney and liver tonic. It is helpful as an analgesic in treating lower back pain and is thought to nourish the bones and tendons.
- Angelica (botanical name, *Angelica* spp.; in Chinese, bai zhi or pai chih). The angelica root is used for its analgesic effect to treat neuralgia, headaches, arthritis, rheumatism, and upset stomachs. It is also an effective tonic for menstrual and blood disorders.
- Arctium (botanical name, *Arctium fructus*; in Chinese, niu bang zi or niu pang tzu). The seed of the arctium is used to relieve inflammatory conditions, swelling, infectious diseases, coughs and sore throats, some types of abscesses, and back pain.
- Arnica (botanical name, *Arnica montana*). The roots and flowers of the arnica plant are used to treat arthritis or sore muscles. It is also effective at healing the inflammation of wounds and bruises. Arnica is often included in liniments. This herb should not be taken internally.
- Astragalus (botanical name, *Astragalus membranaceous*; in Chinese, huang qi). The root of the astragalus is an effective chi tonic that boosts energy and improves the body's resistance to disease. Astragalus is a mild stimulant for general weakness, and it helps fight arthritis, high blood pressure, and heart disease as well as the common cold, allergies, and asthma. It is rich in flavonoids and polysaccharides.

- Bilberry (botanical name, *Vaccinium myrtillus*). The bilberry, or European blueberry, contains flavonoid compounds (called anthocyanosides) that function as potent antioxidants and also decrease capillary fragility and inflammation.

- Black cohosh (botanical name, *Cimicifuga racemosa*). The root of this herb was used for centuries by Native Americans to fight pain and rheumatism. Current research shows that it has anti-inflammatory properties and is effective as a muscle relaxant (to relieve spasms), as a pain reliever, and as a nerve tonic.

- Boswellic acid extract (made from the *Boswellia serrata* tree that is native to India) has antiarthritic and antirheumatic effects, including the ability to reduce inflammation and improve blood supply to the joints. No side effects from boswellic acids have been reported.

- Burdock (botanical name, *Arctium lappa*) is a popular vegetable whose leaves can be applied externally to treat swelling. A root decoction (taken internally) can help treat backache, joint pains (arthritis complaints), bruises, rheumatism, and gout.

- Cayenne pepper (botanical name, *Capsicum frutescens*) contains an active component called capsaicin that fights inflammation and, when applied topically, can stimulate and then block pain fibers. Capsaicin is used as a topical analgesic in several over-the-counter products in the United States. It is also effective in improving digestion and relieving gas.

- Chamomile (*Matricaria chamomilla* [German chamomile] and *Anthemis nobilis* [Roman chamomile]) has a long history of use in treating backache and nervous system and digestive problems. It also has mild sedative properties. Taken internally or applied externally in compresses, chamomile can decrease inflammation and relieve swelling and pain.

- Cinnamon (botanical name, *Cinnamomum cassia*; in Chinese, yueh kuei). Cinnamon twigs (in Chinese, gui zhi) and bark (in Chinese, rou gui) are believed to balance the energy of the lower and upper body, to strengthen circulation, and to warm the body. Cinnamon twigs relieve pains and aches in the back and shoulders. They also calm digestion, induce sweating, and have antiseptic properties. Cinnamon bark functions as an analgesic and a stimulant.

- Devil's claw (botanical name, *Harpagophytum procumbens*) has anti-inflammatory activity and has long been used in the treatment of arthritis and rheumatism. Devil's claw has shown the ability to relieve pain, fight hypertension and rheumatism, relax smooth muscles, and promote joint flexibility.

- Dong quai (botanical name, *Angelica polymorpha*) is an herb greatly respected in China, where it has been used for over two thousand years. It is best known for its use in treating female complaints, including premenstrual syndrome and menopausal symptoms. This root has analgesic, anti-inflammatory, antiarthritis, and anticramping properties.

- Eucalyptus (botanical name, *Eucalyptus globulus*). Oil of eucalyptus with its distinctive camphorlike smell is a popular ingredient in nasal decongestants and topical analgesics. When rubbed on the skin, it appears to be especially effective against arthritis and rheumatism pain, possibly because it brings blood to the area and produces a warm feeling.

- Eucommia (botanical name, *Eucommia ulmoides*; in Chinese, du zhong or tu chung). The eucommia bark is used as a sedative and as an analgesic to alleviate pain in the mid- and lower back. It is said to fortify the bones, tendons, and cartilage and restore injured muscles and bones.

- Fennel (botanical name, *Foeniculum vulgare*; in Chinese, hui shiang) is a popular plant whose roots and seeds are both used in cooking. As a medicinal herb, it fights inflammation and helps decrease joint pain. Fennel is helpful in relieving arthritis and rheumatism pain when rubbed externally.

- Feverfew (botanical name, *Chrysanthemum parthenium*) has a history of use in fighting fever. But it is also effective in fighting headache and pain. This may be because fever-few appears to inhibit prostaglandins involved in inflammation and pain.

- Gardenia (botanical name, *Gardenia florida*; in Chinese, shan zhi zi). The fruit of the gardenia helps decrease fever; relieve headaches, restlessness, and irritability; and detoxify the body. It also functions as an anti-inflammatory agent and can lower blood pressure.

- Garlic (botanical name, *Allium sativum*). Garlic has been used therapeutically for over five thousand years. It is an effective detoxifier, can inhibit inflammation (by modulating the hormones that promote inflammation), and enhances immune function (thereby protecting against infection). Also, garlic strengthens digestion and stimulates metabolism; treats joint and lower back pains, bronchial and lung infections, and urogenital problems; is an immune stimulator; and is excellent in fighting circulatory disorders.

- Gentian (botanical name, *Gentiana lutea*; in Chinese, qin jiao). The gentian root has analgesic and anti-inflammatory effects. It relieves arthritis pain and is often used in herbal combinations containing cinnamon and angelica root to treat tight muscles, arthritis, and rheumatism.

- Gingerroot (botanical name, *Zingiber officinale*; in Chinese, sheng chiang) is used frequently in Chinese cooking, but also has several health applications. Ginger contains a proteolytic enzyme called *zingibain*. Proteolytic enzymes are especially effective at fighting inflammation. Gingerroot has been used to fight arthritis, pain, and inflammation and has a folk history of use for upset stomachs and indigestion.

- Ginseng. There are several types of ginseng including American ginseng (botanical name, *Panax quinquefolius*; in Chinese, xi yang shen) and Asian ginseng (botanical name, *Panax ginseng*; in Chinese, ren shen). Siberian ginseng (botanical name, *Eleutherococcus senticosus*) is not truly a ginseng but has many similar properties. Ginseng has a long history of use in the East and has gained a following in the United States as an energy-enhancing herb. But ginseng can also help the body adapt to stress.

American ginseng is often used to treat nervous exhaustion, fatigue, and sleep disturbances. It is also beneficial in fighting hypertension and in normalizing blood sugar.

One of the most prized tonic herbs in Chinese medicine, Chinese ginseng improves alertness and stamina and decreases the negative effects of mental, emotional, and physical stress. It can increase oxygen utilization, regulate blood sugar, and improve immune function.

■ Hops (botanical name, *Humulus lupulus*), best known as a beer additive, contains lupulinic acid, which decreases the activity of the central nervous system and causes sleep. Hops seems to be an effective pain reliever, sedative, and muscle relaxant. It can also improve digestion.

■ Horse chestnut (botanical name, *Aesculus hippocastanum*). Horse chestnut seeds contain escin, a widely used anti-inflammatory agent. External preparations containing horse chestnut are widely used in Europe.

■ Job's tears (botanical name, *Coix lacryma*; in Chinese, yi yi ren) is a grain that resembles pearl barley. A common food in the East, it relieves bone, tendon, and joint pain, swelling, and inflammation.

■ Kava kava (botanical name, *Piper methysticum*) has been used to promote sleep and induce relaxation. Kava kava may also have an analgesic effect, and it has been prescribed for muscle spasms, rheumatism, gout, insomnia, anxiety, depression, prostate inflammation, and urinary disorders.

■ Licorice root (botanical name, *Glycyrrhiza* spp. in Chinese, gan cao or kan tsao) contains glycyrrhizin, which fights inflammation by inhibiting the synthesis of prostaglandins in much the same way as cortisone. It is often used in herbal combinations because of its sweetness as well as its ability to prolong the effect of other herbs. It is believed to neutralize toxins, improve digestion, relieve muscle spasms, relieve the pain and stiffness of arthritis, lower blood cholesterol, and boost immune function.

- Moutan (botanical name, *Paeonia moutan*; in Chinese, mu dan pi or mu tan pi). The bark of the moutan root is used to fight inflammation, relieve pain, reduce fever, improve circulation, and regulate menstruation. It also has antibacterial activity.
- Mustard (botanical name, *Sinapis alba, S. nigra*). Mustard seeds have a long history of culinary use, but they also appear to be powerful medicine. When used externally in mustard plasters, they can increase the supply of blood to the tissues. They have an anti-inflammatory effect in various conditions, including backache, joint pain, strains, and sprains. *Note:* Do not leave a mustard plaster on the skin for periods longer than ten to fifteen minutes or painful blisters may form. Ointments containing mustard oil are available and used externally much like a mustard plaster to relieve minor pains and aches.
- Notopterygium (in Chinese, qiang huo). The rhizome from the notopterygium relieves joint stiffness and pain, arthritis, rheumatism, and stiff neck.
- Passionflower (botanical name, *Passiflora incarnata*) seems to have a calming effect on the central nervous system. It is often used as a sedative and appears to be helpful in treating anxiety, nerve inflammation, pain, and headaches. It is effective in inducing sleep and calming muscle spasms.
- Red peony (in Chinese, chi shao yao). The root of the red peony is used as an analgesic, as an anti-inflammatory agent, and to fight fever.
- Rehmannia (botanical name, *Rehmannia glutinosa*; in Chinese, shou di huang). The rehmannia root treats mid- and lower back pain. It also reduces fever and is considered a cardiovascular tonic.
- Rhubarb (botanical name, *Rheum palmatum*; in Chinese, da huang). Rhubarb relieves inflammation and pain and promotes blood circulation. The leaves are poisonous, so always use the fruit stalk or rhizome only. *Caution:* Rhubarb is a very effective laxative.
- Rosemary (botanical name, *Rosmarinus officinalis*) is fre-

quently used in cooking but also has a history of use in the treatment of rheumatism and bruises when applied externally in the form of an ointment.

- Saussurea (botanical name, *Saussurea lappa*; in Chinese, mu xiang). The saussurea root is an analgesic that relieves pain and can regulate energy.

- Schizonepeta (botanical name, *Schizonepeta tenuifolia*; in Chinese, jing jie). The schizonepeta seed has analgesic and anti-inflammatory properties. It is effective at treating arthritis and headache as well as colds and fever.

- Siler (botanical name, *Siler divaricatum*; in Chinese, fang feng). Siler root has analgesic properties and relieves muscle and joint pain and aches.

- Skullcap (botanical name, *Scutellaria laterifolia*) has been used as a sedative, pain reliever, and treatment for insomnia. It helps reduce muscle as well as nervous tension.

- St. John's wort (botanical name, *Hypericum perforatum*) has gained a lot of attention lately as a mood elevator and for its soothing effect on injured nerves. But it is also effective when used topically for wounds and bruises.

- Thyme (botanical name, *Thymus vulgaris*) is another popular cooking herb that has a long history of medicinal use. When applied externally, it appears effective in relieving pain and inflammation.

- Turmeric (botanical name, *Curcuma longa*; in Chinese, chiang huang) is an herb popularly used in the Ayurvedic medicine of India. An active ingredient in turmeric called *curcumin* is used internally as a digestive aid, an anti-inflammatory agent, an analgesic, and an antioxidant. Externally, it may help relieve arthritis pain.

- Valerian (botanical name, *Valerian officinalis*) is often used as a sleep aid because of its sedative action. It is effective in treating nervous tension, anxiety, muscle pain, and headache.

- White willow (botanical name, *Salix alba*). White willow bark has been used for centuries as a pain reliever because it is a natural source of salicin (a precursor of our modern aspirin). White willow suppresses prostaglandin production, reduces inflammation, and relieves muscle strains and pain from injuries, rheumatism, or arthritis.

- Wild cherry (botanical name, *Prunus virginiana*). The bark from the wild cherry was used by several Native American tribes as a sedative and pain reliever and to calm nervous excitability.
- Wild yam (botanical name, *Dioscorea villosa*) contains a phytochemical called *diosgenin* that has demonstrated anti-inflammatory effects. This may be why wild yam has historically been used to treat rheumatism.
- Wintergreen (botanical name, *Gaultheria procumbens*), when used externally as oil of wintergreen, is effective in relieving body aches and pains.
- Yarrow (*Achillea millefolium*) is known to have a calming effect and has anti-inflammatory properties.

Herbal Combination Principle

In TCM, combinations of herbs are usually used to obtain the optimal therapeutic result. Most often, the herbal combination will contain six to twelve different herbs, but the number of herbs will vary by formula. Herbs are combined for a number of reasons:

1. Each herb has its own distinctive biochemical properties, and combining several herbs can have a synergistic action. The herbs work better together than any one herb could work separately.
2. Combining herbs can speed their therapeutic effect.
3. Combining herbs can decrease the possibility of side effects and toxicity that may occur if large amounts of a single herb were taken. Sometimes, one herb can neutralize any toxic effects of large quantities of another herb.

Herbal formulas used in TCM should not be treated lightly. Chinese herbal formulas can have serious side effects.

Don't believe the old adage that if a little bit is good, more is better. It won't work with Chinese herbal formulas. The amounts noted in this book have been taken from reputable sources. But don't take chances. Work with a well-trained and skilled Chinese herbal practitioner. Also, one herb or one herbal combination does not fit all; there are individual differences. Each person is unique, and each person has a special pattern of disharmony and harmony. Therefore, unique proportions and combinations of herbs must be found for each person. Two people may complain of similar symptoms, but it is the underlying imbalance that must be treated.

If you self-diagnose your condition inaccurately and use TCM formulas and other OTC products without consultation, you could hurt, rather than help, yourself.

Chinese Herbal Combination Formulas

Over the centuries, Chinese herbalists have developed certain unique formulas to treat arthritis, rheumatism, and other conditions causing inflammation, swelling, and back pain. The following patent formulas are six of the most commonly used Chinese herbal combinations. You can find these combinations in most Chinese herbal shops. Use these formulas as instructed on the label.

Combination #1: Bear-Gall Sport Injury Pill (hsiung tan tieh tah wan) This combination is especially effective for inflammation from traumatic injuries, severe bruises, swelling, and sprains. This formula is popular in China for injuries from martial arts training and sports. It encourages rapid healing of injured blood vessels and more rapid breakup of stagnated blood; it also stimulates blood flow, dispels heat, and decreases swelling.

Ingredients

amomum fruit	curcuma root
angelica	inula root
bear gall	pseudoginseng root
carthamus	rhubarb

Combination #2: Ginseng and Deer-Horn Pills (jen shen lu jung wan) This formula is effective as a restorative tonic after extended and chronic pain and illness (such as lower back pain, lumbago, and sciatica), fatigue, poor appetite, poor memory, and insomnia. It improves immune, cerebral, and sex function. It tones the kidneys and gives energy to the kidneys' yin and yang and to the spleen.

Ingredients

achyranthes	ginseng
angelica	honey
astragalus	longan fruit
deer horn	morinda root
eucommia	

Combination #3: Male Treasure (nan bao capsules) This formula gives relief from lower back pain, chronic fatigue, and indigestion and is a good geriatric tonic for men. It relieves kidney yang deficiency from aging and improves endocrine function. It is a popular and potent male tonic for kidney energy, blood energy, and spleen energy and for premature ejaculation, impotence, loss of sex drive, and insufficient erection.

Ingredients

achyranthes	epimedium
aconite	eucommia
angelica	ginseng
astragalus	licorice
atractylodes	lycium
cinnamon	morinda root
cistanche	ophiopogon root
cornus fruit	paeonia root
curculigo	poria cocos
cuscuta	psorelea
cynomorium	rehmannia
deer horn	rubus
dipsacus	scrophularia

dog kidney	sea horse
donkey kidney	trigonella
donkey skin glue	

Combination #4: Clematis and Stephania Combination (shu ching huo hsieh tang)

Combination #4: Clematis and Stephania Combination (shu ching huo hsieh tang) This combination is effective in treating muscular rheumatism, arthritis, myofascial pain syndrome, fibromyalgia, sciatica, and neuralgia. It is good for migratory aches such as back pain and leg pain, especially during the night. The combination contains seventeen herbs and is used with people who have difficulty recovering from pain and illness and those with a weak constitution.

Ingredients

achyranthes	licorice
angelica	paeonia
atractylodes	persica
citrus	qianghuo
clematis	rehmannia
cnidium	siler
gentiana	stephania
ginger	tang kuei
hoelen	

Dosage: Take two or three capsules two or three times per day between meals and on an empty stomach for two to three months for lasting effects. It is possible to experience pain relief as quickly as one hour after taking this herbal combination. But continue taking it for permanent results. *Note:* If stomach distress develops and persists over a few days, discontinue the herbal combination.

Combination #5: Coix Combination (i yi jen tang)

Combination #5: Coix Combination (i yi jen tang) This combination is effective against muscular rheumatism, myofascial pain syndrome, fibromyalgia, rheumatoid arthritis, osteoarthritis (especially in the early stages), fever, back pain, swelling, sciatica, lumbago, and generalized muscle and joint pain. Coix combination is also used to improve digestion and for improved constitution.

Ingredients

atractylodes	licorice
cinnamon	paeonia
coix	tang kuei

Dosage: Take coix combination as either a tea (drink two or three times every day) or in capsule form, taking two or three capsules two or three times a day between meals on an empty stomach for two to three months for lasting effects. It is possible to experience pain relief as quickly as one hour after taking the remedy. However, continue taking the herbal combination for permanent relief. *Note:* If stomach distress develops and persists over a few days, discontinue the combination.

Combination #6: Arthritis and Joint Pain Chinese Herbal Combination This combination decreases joint pain from both rheumatoid arthritis and osteoarthritis and from backache, rheumatism, and gout. It also fights inflammation and neuralgia.

Ingredients

angelica	dandelion
burdock	garden nettle
catmint	ginger
Chinese cinnamon	marigold
(cassia)	sage
coriander	stinging nettle

This combination may be taken internally in the capsular form. However, seek the consultation of a well-trained herbal physician before beginning a self-treatment program.

Dosage: Take as indicated on the label and between meals on an empty stomach. Continue taking the herbal combination for two to three months for lasting effects.

WHERE CAN YOU BUY CHINESE HERBS AND HERBAL FORMULAS?

You can buy Chinese herbal formulas at your local health food store or at herbal shops that sell Chinese herbal formulas. Most large cities have shops specializing in Chinese herbal formulas. You can also obtain the formulas from the following companies:

Brion Herbs Corporation
9250 Jeronimo Road
Irvine, CA 92718
Tel: (714) 587-1238
Fax: (714) 587-1260

Dragon River Herbal
P.O. Box 74
Ojo Caliente, NM 87549
Tel/Fax: (505) 583-2118

Golden State Herbs, Inc.
P. O. Box 810
Occidental, CA 95465

Haussmann's Pharmacy
534-536 West Girard Avenue
Philadelphia, PA 19123-1444

Health Concerns
2415 Mariner Square Drive, #3
Alameda, CA 94501
Tel: 1-800-233-9355

Indiana Botanical Gardens, Inc.
P.O. Box 5
Hammond, IN 46325

K'an Herb Company
2425 Porter Street
Soquel, CA 95073
Fax: (408) 479-9118

Kanpo Formulas
P. O. Box 60279
Sacramento, CA 95860
Tel: (916) 487-9044

Kwan Yin Chinese Herb Co., Inc.
P.O. Box 18617
Spokane, WA 99208

Mayway Trading Company
780 Broadway
San Francisco, CA 95073
Tel: (415) 788-3646

Nature's Herb Co.
281 Ellis Street
San Francisco, CA 94102

Nu-Life Nutrition
871 Beatty Street
Vancouver, BC, Canada

Vital Herb
Everyoung Herbs Ltd.
1850 South Sepulveda Boulevard, Suite 203
Los Angeles, CA 90025
Tel: (310) 479-8862
Fax: (310) 479-4466

Zand Herbal Formulas
P.O. Box 2039
Boulder, CO 80306
Tel: 1-800-800-0405

RAPID REVIEW

- Nutritional stress places an imbalance on the entire body that can manifest as muscle tension, leading to spasms and pain.
- Improving your body's biochemistry can go a long way toward improving your body's overall health, as well as improving the function of nerves, muscles, tendons, and ligaments; strengthening bones; and reducing pain. You can improve your biochemistry by:
    - Detoxifying regularly by eliminating your exposure to external toxins, increasing your water intake, and juice fasting.
    - Eating a proper diet. Follow the USDA's food pyramid and include lots of enzyme-rich fresh foods.
    - Taking supplements, including vitamins, minerals, enzymes, herbs, and other nutrients.

Nine

Physical
Healing Secrets

lthough balancing your emotional and nutritional
status is important in your fight against back pain, it
often is not enough. Unless you also balance the
disharmony in your physical health and strengthen your
body, you will not recover from back pain. There are several
physical healing secrets that can return you to health and
help prevent future back problems. One of the best ways to
recover from, as well as to prevent, back pain is physical
exercise. But even exercise may not be enough. Fortunately,
there are a number of physical techniques that, in addition to
the emotional and nutritional techniques discussed earlier in
this book, can help you recover from back pain. This chapter
will explain how you can help yourself using a number of
techniques. Some are widely practiced in this country; others
are more popular in the East but are extremely effective and
becoming increasingly popular in the Western world.

Both Traditional Chinese Medicine (TCM) and Western
medicine recognize the need for exercise to rehabilitate the
back, prevent back pain, improve circulation, and increase
vitality. But your exercise time can also give you an opportunity to meditate, turn your thoughts inward, visualize your
back pain leaving, and increase your energy level.

Some exercises, especially yoga, qi gong, and tai chi, are particularly beneficial for building up, rather than depleting, energy. These exercises (which will be explained later in this chapter) not only improve muscle strength, posture, and oxygen intake through body movement but also have positive effects on various body functions as well as on the emotions and are important for long-term well-being and health.

EXERCISE

In today's fast-paced society, staying healthy is only possible through a balanced lifestyle, of which physical exercise is an important part. The benefits of exercise are many.

1. Exercise improves muscle tone, increases lean muscle tissue, and helps strengthen the muscles that support your back.
2. Exercise helps you to overcome low back pain and "lubricates" spinal disks.
3. Physical exercise releases endorphins, which are morphinelike hormones in the brain. These hormones produce a sense of well-being in the body and cause us to actually feel better. You will feel happier, refreshed, and more relaxed—possibly even after your first or second workout. You'll have more positive feelings about your life and your health and will be better able to deal with the stresses of everyday life.
4. Exercise increases circulation, thus improving the delivery of oxygen and nutrients to all the tissues of the body. Increased circulation allows for more efficient elimination of any metabolic waste products.
5. Exercise strengthens bones. As we age, our bones lose density and weaken (a condition called *osteoporosis*). This is particularly serious in older women. However, a regular exercise program can decrease the rate of bone loss and can sometimes even stop or reverse the effects of osteoporosis. Further, those who continue physical activity into their golden years are less likely to suffer from osteoporosis.
6. Exercise can help you lose weight and keep it off. It

decreases fat stores and helps you burn calories, even when at rest. Excess weight is often the cause of back pain.

7. Exercise can also help strengthen the heart and lungs. It can help you reduce your blood pressure and also control a number of health conditions, including coronary heart disease, hypertension, and non-insulin-dependent diabetes. In fact, if you are physically active, you are almost half as likely to develop coronary heart disease as people who do not exercise regularly.

8. Exercise can increase your energy level and help you fight fatigue.

9. Exercise increases your mental capacity and may even improve your IQ! Improved mental capacity may also improve the flow of nerve messages, as well as your level of coordination, since it improves your muscular balance. If your back hurts, you will probably sit, stand, or walk differently to avoid pain. But this can lead to muscular imbalance, something that can be improved and stabilized with exercise.

10. Exercise makes you look younger and fights the ravages of aging. Improved circulation means healthier, younger-looking skin.

11. Exercise can give you more restful and continuous sleep.

12. Exercise can improve your sex life. In fact, those who exercise regularly report greater sexual activity and increased sexual desire.

There are actually four main exercise categories in the rehabilitation and prevention of back pain. These four categories are the cross-patterning technique; stretching and flexibility exercises; muscle-strengthening exercises; and aerobic exercises for cardiovascular endurance. This chapter will explain the benefits of these exercises and give you clear and concise directions explaining how to perform them.

Other beneficial exercises explained in this chapter include yoga, qi gong, and tai chi. These exercises can help strengthen you physically while also improving your emotional state.

Physical modalities (including ice and heat), manual techniques (such as massage), and orthotics (including braces, corsets, and foot supports) can all help relieve back pain and return your back to health. These techniques and devices are discussed later in this chapter.

When Should You Begin Exercising?

If you have just suffered an acute traumatic injury, several days of rest may be helpful. Check with your doctor to be sure. But rest is usually not recommended beyond a few days and may actually delay your recovery. In fact, extended bed rest can result in numerous unhealthy and unpleasant effects, including stiffness, loss of strength, decreased cardiopulmonary endurance, contractures, and metabolic changes. This is because the inflammatory processes that result from injury can cause congestion in the tissues.

A recent study on low back pain conducted in the United Kingdom found that advice to continue ordinary activities and stay active resulted in a more rapid return to work, fewer recurrent problems, and less chronic disability.[1]

Generally speaking, exercises should be avoided for the first few days to a week after an injury. After a few days, mild stretching can be initiated. After your pain has diminished (in one to two weeks), and with your physician's approval, you can usually begin mild aerobic and strengthening exercises. Tailor the exercises explained in this chapter to fit your individual needs. Begin at your own comfort level.

Exercises in this book have been chosen because they are simple and easy to learn. They are designed for individuals who are physically fit and in good health, but they are not intended as a substitute for medical counseling. Only perform those exercises that are easy to do and are painless. Not all exercises are suitable for all people, and this or any other exercise program may cause injury. If any exercise causes you pain, stop and don't do that specific exercise. Never force or strain to perform an exercise. Remember, the first step in treating your back pain is to cause no harm. Consult with your physician before beginning this or any other exercise plan.

The Rules of Exercising

1. Exercise every day for twenty-five to thirty minutes without exception. Develop a schedule, and reserve special time every day to exercise. For variety, you can break up the program, trying different exercises. Exercise just after rising in the morning and/or just before going to bed.

2. Almost everyone is able to do some type of exercise, whether it's simply deep breathing, walking, stretching, or more active exercise such as jogging or bicycling.

3. Begin with the cross-patterning exercises explained in this chapter and progress to the stretching and flexibility exercises. Mild stretching exercises help increase circulation, remove toxins, and begin to improve flexibility. Use mild stretching exercises and mild yoga exercises in a supine or prone position. Then tackle the strengthening exercises and finally the aerobic exercises.

   In most cases, back pain is minimized when you are lying down because there is less force of gravity exerted on the back and spine. However, the weight of gravity increases as you sit and then stand. Therefore, when recovering from back pain, first use the exercises in this book that are performed while lying down. Then graduate to those performed in a sitting position, and ultimately to those performed while standing. In addition, the tai chi exercises, explained later in this chapter, are performed while standing and require a certain amount of muscular strength and balance as well as constant movement. Therefore, tai chi should be chosen last in the continuum. However, tai chi is an excellent exercise program and way of life.

4. Initially, you may experience some minimal soreness if you haven't exercised in awhile. But exercising to the point of excessive stiffness, soreness, and fatigue won't help your condition. "No pain, no gain" is definitely not in the program. Extreme pain is a warning sign that you're overdoing it. Give yourself a few days of rest if you experience moderate to severe soreness, particularly in or around the joints. Overdoing it is the most

common mistake people make in exercising, and it is the most frequent reason people quit exercising. After the soreness subsides, gradually return to your exercise regimen. You should feel great once your body adjusts.

5. Wear comfortable, loose, and breathable clothing.
6. Exercise may be more fun if you enlist a friend who can help you keep motivated.
7. Keep a progress chart so that you can see where you started and how far you've come. Note how you feel during and after exercising. Eventually, you'll see an improvement.
8. If a back specialist is supervising your back care, follow his or her directions.
9. In addition, if you have a serious chronic condition, such as a cardiovascular condition, or have any major risk factors for coronary disease (such as diabetes, high blood pressure, cigarette smoking, obesity, or a family history of heart disease), consult your physician before beginning any exercise program.

Level of Difficulty for Exercises

The exercises in the following program have varying levels of difficulty. For example, level 1 exercises (the beginning level) are the easiest to perform, would be the first type of exercise you should attempt as your back pain decreases, and are performed lying down. On the other hand, level 6 exercises are the most difficult to perform, require the greatest amount of dexterity, endurance, and coordination, and are performed while standing (but may include other postures).

These levels are general guidelines only. There can be individual differences. What may be easy for you to perform may be more difficult for someone else. Remember, if any exercise causes pain, stop immediately. *Note:* All of these exercises can be performed in conjunction with breathing exercises and meditation.

Table 9.1 describes my six levels of exercising for better health, more energy, increased weight loss, decreased back pain, and a longer life.

Table 9.1

EXERCISE LEVELS OF DIFFICULTY

LEVEL OF DIFFICULTY	EXERCISES	WHEN TO ATTEMPT THIS LEVEL
1	Those performed while lying on your back or stomach, including those that involve stretching, as well as some of the beginning yoga exercises	As back pain begins to decrease (the emphasis should be on stretching, rather than strengthening)
2	Those exercises performed while sitting, including those that involve stretching, as well as some of the beginning yoga exercises	When you can sit or lie without pain (the emphasis should be on stretching, not strengthening)
3	Those stretching exercises performed while standing, including warm-up or loosening-up exercises, such as those in tai chi and tae-bo	When you can stand in an upright position without pain (again, the emphasis should be on stretching, not strengthening)

(Continued)

Table 9.1 *(Continued)*

LEVEL OF DIFFICULTY	EXERCISES	WHEN TO ATTEMPT THIS LEVEL
4	Qi gong; tai chi (the beginning movements); yoga (increased flexibility exercises); tae-bo (slow movement of complete exercises); aerobics (beginning)	When you are able perform the exercises in levels 1, 2, and 3 without pain and have more movement and greater endurance and are more flexible (these exercises begin to strengthen muscles)
5	Tai chi (full program); tae-bo (increased speed of movement); increased level of aerobics, such as stair stepper	When you are able to perform level 4 exercises without pain
6	Tae-bo by Billy Blanks, combination of dance boxing and karate (full speed); tai chi (full program); yoga (full program)	When you are able to perform level 5 exercises without pain and have the endurance to perform more strenuous activity

THE EXERCISES
Cross-Patterning/Cross-Crawl

When we crawl, creep, and walk normally, we don't think about what we're doing, we just do it. But for the body to function and walk, stand, sit, or move in a coordinated fashion, the brain must send clear messages to various parts of the body. Just as all cylinders must work in sync in your car, so must various body parts work together for coordinated movement. If your muscles aren't functioning properly, as often happens with back pain, they will begin to atrophy and weaken, and nerve transmission will be decreased, leading to an imbalance in the body. A good way to improve nerve transmission is through cross-crawl. As mentioned in chapter 4, the cross-crawl technique was originally developed by Temple Fay, M.D., and continued by Glenn Doman to help brain-injured children. However, it can also help correct body imbalances because it apparently acts to train (or retrain) us to correctly process the messages from the brain regarding movement. The cross-crawl technique is excellent not only for brain-injured children but for everyone.

Cross-crawl is the term used by Fay and Doman in treating brain-injured children, and the technique involves working with the child facedown and in a prone position. *Cross-patterning* is a term used in applied kinesiology, with the individual lying in a supine position, on the knees, or in an upright position and walking. All positions involve similar nerve functions, but the terms *cross-crawl* and *cross-patterning* mainly refer to the position the individual takes in performing the exercises. That is, cross-crawl is performed lying facedown, while cross-patterning is performed lying on the back, on the hands and knees, or in an upright position and walking.

At varying times during his rehabilitation, my son David's back muscles were flaccid, spastic, or rigid. This caused a great deal of back muscle imbalance and resulting back pain. Relaxing the spastic and rigid muscles using massage and cross-patterning, while also stretching and strengthening the weak and flaccid muscles, helped balance the muscles and relieved his back pain. Because the brain controls information to and from the torso, arms, and legs, a properly functioning brain and spinal cord are essential for coordination between arms, legs, and torso. David experienced less and less back pain the more his balance and coordination improved.

I don't know whether David would have recovered without cross-crawl/cross-patterning. What I do know is that David *did* recover and *did* become an outstanding athlete and student. Cross-crawl/cross-patterning has been shown to improve mobility, manual and tactile competence, visual and auditory competence, and language skills—even in those having normal brain function.

Further, I have used cross-patterning with many children and adults afflicted with back pain and decreased mobility. The success of the technique seems to be influenced by a number of variables, such as the severity of the injury, the location of the injury, the time spent each day using the cross-patterning technique, and the age and physical condition of the patient. However, cross-patterning's success is not limited to those suffering from back pain due to injury. Whatever the cause of your back pain, cross-patterning can help. By improving brain function and therefore the transmission of messages throughout the body, you can improve neuromusculoskeletal coordination.

The cross-patterning exercises can be performed lying on your back, kneeling on your hands and knees, standing, or lying on your stomach.

Cross-Patterning on Your Back (Level 1)
- Lie on your back with your legs extended and relaxed, shoulder-width apart. Your arms should be at your sides.
- While lifting your left arm up over your head, turn your head to the left and bring your right knee up to your chest.
- Then lower your left arm and right leg and raise your right arm over your head, turning your head to the right and lifting your left knee to your chest.
- Repeat with the left arm, then the right arm, and so on.
- Movement should be smooth and continuous.

- Do this exercise at least 4 times daily (upon rising, mid-morning, mid-afternoon, and before retiring) for 5 minutes at each session.
- *Note:* If the evening cross-patterning is too stimulating and causes loss of sleep, skip the evening session.
- Athletes can benefit by performing this technique just before and after a workout or a competitive event.
- Some people find it easier to perform this technique lying on their stomach.

Cross-Patterning Diagonal Reach on Your Hands and Knees (Level 2)

- Begin on your hands and knees on a firm surface, such as the floor.
- Slowly extend your right arm out in front of you, turning your head to the right and straightening your left leg out behind you. At this point, your body is being supported by your left arm and your right knee.
- Hold for 5 seconds.
- Switch sides (left arm and right leg).

Cross-Patterning Standing Up (Level 3)

- Stand upright.
- Raise your right arm above your head while turning your head to the right and lifting your left knee as high as possible.
- Repeat using the left arm and the right leg, turning your head to the left.
- Make movements continuous and flowing from one side to the other.

For individuals with severe back pain who are unable to perform this technique unassisted, cross-crawl/cross-patterning can be administered by three adults. One adult turns the head, another moves the right leg and arm, and the third moves the left leg and arm. The patterns must be performed rhythmically and smoothly at all levels.

The purpose of this section on cross-crawl/cross-patterning has been to give you an introduction to the technique. For further information and materials on cross-patterning, contact:

The Institutes for the Achievement of Human Potential
8801 Stenton Avenue
Philadelphia, PA 19038-8397
Tel: (215) 233-2050

Stretching and Flexibility Exercises

General stretching and flexibility exercises can be used by all back pain sufferers to eliminate back pain. Whether you have severe pain due to a structural instability or mild pain because of chronic fatigue, these exercises can improve your condition and can be performed without fear of harming your back if you do them according to instructions.

Muscle tension is one of your body's automatic physical reactions to stress. This muscle tension can result in back pain. Stretching is a simple way to combat this stress, to relax muscle tension, and to relieve the symptoms of back pain. Don't allow the stress to build up. It takes only a few minutes to do these exercises at work (at lunch or coffee breaks), at home, at play, or whenever tension begins to rear its ugly head.

TIPS FOR STRETCHING EXERCISES

- Perform the exercises twice daily (morning and evening) when you first begin the program. As you progress, perform them once daily to remain flexible.
- Dress warmly and comfortably in loose-fitting clothes made from soft fabrics. Tight pants, large buttons, belts, buckles, and clothes with no stretch can all inhibit your exercises.
- Perform all the exercises on a firm, flat surface, preferably an exercise mat or a towel placed on a carpeted floor.
- Exercises should be done carefully, with a minimum of stress and strain. Stretching requires patience and concentration to make sure you are following the proper technique. Stretch gradually until you feel resistance, using your own body weight and gravity to define your stretching zone.
- Stretch slowly. Rome wasn't built in a day. Don't rush through

the stretches and don't bounce. Bouncy or fast movements can increase your risk of injury. Perform your stretches with controlled and slow movements. Stretch only to a point beyond which would cause discomfort.

- Let your breathing come from your diaphragm. Take three deep breaths for relaxation and begin with easy, gentle movements. With each breath, your stomach, not your shoulders and rib cage, should rise and fall. Abdominal breathing helps lower blood pressure, lessens muscular tension, and encourages relaxation.
- Stretching and flexibility exercises are not competitive sports. At first, you may not be as flexible as others, but don't be discouraged. Each person's flexibility can vary greatly. You may not improve immediately; it may take a while, but if you stick with the program and enjoy it at your own pace, you *will* improve.
- Visualize your muscles relaxing, gradually and slowly, as you close your eyes and feel your muscles.
- Pain does not equal gain. Never stretch to the point of pain.
- Be patient. It will take about three weeks before you can perform the exercises comfortably. Gradually increase the number of repetitions until you are able to complete ten of them without excessive discomfort.
- If you have any questions about stretching exercises, ask a back specialist.

Best Time for Stretching Just as a dog or cat stretches as it awakens, so should you begin every day with a stretch. At work, stretching can help you relieve nervous tension and can keep you mentally alert. You should always stretch after you have been standing or sitting for a long time. You can stretch anytime during the day—while watching television or driving in your car. But be careful not to stretch cold muscles to their maximum.

The following stretching and flexibility program begins by stretching your entire body, then mildly stretching specific muscles of the body.

Stretching Exercise #1: Full-Body Stretch (Level 3) This
exercise stretches the muscles of your spine and will warm up
and energize your entire body.

- Stand with your arms at your sides. Point your toes forward
  and stand with your weight mainly on the balls of your feet.
- Lift your arms into the air, over and behind your head as
  far as possible. Stretch your arms and reach for the sky.
- Hold for 10 seconds.
- Slowly lower your arms and relax.
- Repeat 5 times.

Stretching Exercise #2: Lateral Neck Stretch (Level 2)
This exercise stretches the muscles of the neck and can
increase their flexibility.

- Stand or sit up straight.
- Gently bend your head to the right, as though you were
  trying to put your head on your shoulder.
- Hold for 5 seconds, then return to center.
- Then bend your head to the left and hold for 5 seconds.
- Repeat 5 times on each side.

Stretching Exercise #3: Head Rotation (Level 1) This exercise stretches the muscles of the neck and can increase their
flexibility.

- Turn your head as far as you can to the right, without
  causing pain.
- Hold this position while exhaling for 10 seconds.
- Repeat the same rotation to the left.
- Repeat this exercise 5 times.

Stretching Exercise #4: Shoulder Shrug (Level 2) This
exercise helps relax the muscles of the neck, shoulders, and
upper back.

- Sit or stand comfortably.
- Lift your shoulders.

- Slowly let your shoulders relax.
- Repeat this exercise at least 5 times or whenever you have neck, shoulder, or upper back pain.

Stretching Exercise #5: Shoulder and Upper Back Stretch (Level 3) This exercise stretches the lower back and abdominal muscles and relaxes the back muscles.

- Stand arm's length away from a wall or other strong vertical surface.
- Place both hands shoulder-width apart on the wall.
- Move your feet backward from the wall until they are about 3 feet from the wall.
- Keep your feet directly below your hips.
- Tip your pelvis slightly, bending at the knees, and arch your back.
- Hold for 5 seconds.
- Repeat 5 times.

Stretching Exercise #6: Upper Back Stretch (Level 2) This exercise stretches the muscles of the upper back and shoulders.

- Bring your left arm across your chest, with the elbow flexed and the left hand open and reaching over your right shoulder.
- With the right hand, grasp the left elbow.
- While turning your head and looking to the right, use the right hand to pull the left elbow farther across your chest. Do not force.
- Hold for 5 to 10 seconds.
- Take a deep breath and relax.
- Repeat this procedure on the right side.
- Repeat 5 times.

Stretching Exercise #7: Back Extension (Level 3) This exercise stretches the muscles of the chest and abdomen.

- Stand comfortably and place your hands on the back of your hips.

- Slowly and gently bend your upper body backward.
- Move back only as far as you feel comfortable.
- Continue to support your back with your hands.
- Hold for 5 seconds.
- To return to an upright position, tighten your abdominal muscles, bring your head forward, and push with your arms and hands.
- Repeat 5 times.

Stretching Exercise #8: Standing Side Bend (Level 3) This exercise stretches the muscles in the sides.

- Stand with hands on hips.
- Bend—only at the waist—slowly and to the right side.
- Do not tip the pelvis.
- Keep knees slightly bent.
- Hold for 5 seconds.
- Return to the upright position.
- Repeat 5 times.
- Repeat by bending to the left side.

Stretching Exercise #9: "Chair" Lower Back and Total Spinal Stretch (Level 3) I call this exercise "chair" because you are actually forming a chair with your body. It is an excellent exercise to stretch the muscles of your lower back and tighten your abdominal muscles. It is also excellent for tension relaxation.

- Stand with your back up against a wall or other firm vertical structure. Your feet should be shoulder-width apart, and your heels should be against the wall.
- Try to make contact between the wall and your head, midback, and lower back.
- With short, alternating steps, slide your right, then left foot away from the wall while continuing to maintain contact between the wall and your back.
- As you move out from the wall, bend your knees and gradually slide your back down the wall until you reach a chairlike position. Slide as far, but no more, than your

leg strength will allow you. While sliding, tighten your legs and abdominal muscles and tip the lower portion of your pelvis forward. Maintain contact between your back and the wall.

- Now, with your head, midback, and lower back still in contact with the wall, and your chin tucked in, begin to move your feet slowly and easily back to the wall.
- When your feet have reached the wall, visualize your body's posture at this time. A full-length mirror can be an excellent help. Look in the mirror: observe and internalize your posture.
- Walk away from the wall, trying to maintain the posture you have felt, visualized, seen, and experienced. Try to keep your knees relaxed, your pelvis slightly tipped forward, and your abdominal muscles firm and tight.

The more frequently you repeat this exercise, the better your posture will be. The end result is decreased back pain.

Note: An extension of the chair exercise while you are leaning against the wall is to progressively tighten the abdominal muscles and to continue flattening your back from the tailbone through the lower back and up the midback in a rolling fashion.

Stretching Exercise #10: Passive Back Stretch (Level 1)
This exercise stretches and relaxes the muscles of your lower back and is great at relieving lower back pain.

- Lie on the floor with your legs on a chair or resting on pillows. Your arms should be at your sides. If you wish, place a cervical pillow under your neck.
- Relax, pressing your lower back against the floor. Try to feel your tailbone tilting forward, and progressively feel each individual vertebra coming in contact with the floor.
- Rest in this position for 1 to 2 minutes.
- Relax.
- Repeat 5 times or as often as you wish.

Stretching Exercise #11: Hamstring Stretch (Level 3) This exercise stretches the hamstring muscles in the back of your leg. Tight and therefore shortened hamstrings can cause muscular imbalance in your lower back.

- Stand facing a wall.
- Place your hands against the wall at about eye level.
- Your right foot should be 2 to $2^1/_2$ feet behind the left foot.
- Both of your heels should be on the floor.
- Slowly lean forward until you feel a pull in your right leg's hamstring muscle.
- Hold for about 5 to 10 seconds.
- Slowly stand up straight, decreasing the pull in your right calf.
- Repeat the exercise 5 times.
- Repeat the exercise with your left foot 2 to $2^1/_2$ feet behind the right.

Stretching Exercise #12: Squat Stretch (Level 3) This exercise stretches the back muscles of your entire spine.

- Take a squat position.
- Put your hands on your knees.
- Bend your head and body, lowering your body until your chest and thighs are parallel to each other and to the floor (extend your arms forward, if needed, for balance).
- Bend your head as far forward as possible.
- Hold this position for 10 seconds.
- Gradually return to a neutral position by gently pushing upward with your hands and arms.
- Repeat 5 times.

Stretching Exercise #13: Frog Leg (Level 1) This exercise stretches your hip muscles and the muscles that run along the inside of your thighs.
- Lie on your back with your knees bent.
- Relax your knees and allow the knees to fall to the sides, nearly touching the floor.
- Hold the knees open for 5 seconds.

- Bring the knees together in the middle.
- Repeat the exercise 10 times.

Stretching Exercise #14: Pelvic Tilt (Level 1) This exercise stretches the abdominal muscles and those of the lower back.

- Lie on your back with your knees bent 90 degrees and feet flat on the floor.
- Slowly take a deep breath in and then slowly exhale for 5 seconds as you tighten your abdominal and buttock muscles, pressing your lower back against the floor.
- Relax.
- Repeat 10 times.

Stretching Exercise #15: Knee Pull (Level 1) This exercise stretches your back muscles and helps to limber up a stiff back and hips.

- Lie on your back.
- Tip your pelvis forward and tighten your abdominal muscles.
- Bend your knees and slowly draw them up to your chest using your abdominal muscles.
- Clasp your hands firmly around your knees and pull toward your chest.
- Hold for 5 seconds.
- Gradually straighten your legs as you slowly relax your abdominal muscles.
- Repeat 10 times.

Stretching Exercise #16: Lower Back Flexion Stretch (Level 3) This exercise stretches your entire back (especially the lower back).

- Stand erect but relaxed.
- Hunch forward, dropping your arms in front of your body.
- Your knees should be slightly bent.
- Tip your pelvis forward and tighten your abdominal muscles while you relax your back muscles.

- Let your hands drop as far as they can.
- Bend your head forward and drop your shoulders until you feel a pull in your lower back.
- Hold for 5 seconds.
- Slowly return to an upright position and relax.
- Repeat 10 times.

Stretching Exercise #17: Dog and Cat (Level 2) This exercise increases flexibility in the back and abdominal muscles.

- Start on your hands and knees with your torso parallel to the floor and your back straight.
- Looking up toward the ceiling, lift your head as high as possible and curve your back downward. Hold for 5 seconds.
- Then lower your head and arch your lower back toward the ceiling (much as a cat arches its back while hissing). Hold for 5 seconds.
- Return to the starting position.
- Repeat 10 times.

Stretching Exercise # 18: Bent-Knee Stretch (Level 1) This exercise stretches the hip and back muscles, increasing their flexibility.

- Lie on your back with both knees bent and feet flat on the floor.
- Pull your left knee to your chest.
- Breathe deeply and hold for 10 seconds.
- Lower your left knee.
- Pull your right knee to your chest and hold for 10 seconds.
- Lower your right knee.
- Repeat 10 times.

Stretching Exercise # 19: Straight-Leg Stretch (Level 1) This exercise stretches the hamstring muscles and improves back flexibility.

- Lie on your back with both knees bent and feet flat on the floor.
- Straighten your left leg and try to raise it as high as possible, with comfort.
- Hold for 5 seconds.
- Return to the starting position.
- Raise your right leg as high as possible.
- Hold for 5 seconds.
- Repeat this exercise 5 times.

Stretching Exercise #20: Grass Drill (Level 4) As your back improves, this exercise is excellent for improving balance and back flexibility.

- Perform this exercise on grass or a large, flat surface.
- As you step forward on your right leg, bend down, and with your left hand reach for an imaginary object on the floor.
- Return upright.
- Then step forward on your left leg, bend down, and with your right hand reach for an imaginary object on the floor.
- Return to an upright position and repeat this exercise for 40 steps.
- Initially do this exercise slowly. As you become more comfortable with the exercise, you can increase the pace to a trot or a slow run. Also, you can alter the pace (fast, slow) for variety.

Note: I have successfully used this exercise (an extension of cross-patterning) for world-class athletes, as well as weekend warriors and brain-damaged children.

MUSCLE-STRENGTHENING EXERCISES
Weak muscles can cause back instability and increase your risk of suffering from muscle spasms, disk degeneration, pinched nerves, vertebral subluxations, pain, and other problems. Therefore, back muscles must not only be stretched but also strengthened in order to keep spinal balance. But,

strangely, weak back muscles are less frequently a cause of lower back pain than weak abdominal muscles. In fact, the spine is supported from the front by various muscle groups. This support is especially important to the health of the lower back. Muscles of the abdomen must be strong enough to compress the organs of the body snugly against the spinal column if lower back pain is to be avoided. Strong abdominal muscles help to strengthen the lower back and hold the lower spine upright, keeping the spine from curving excessively forward.

Further, there is a subtle but constant give and take involving various muscles in the body. For example, the muscles of the abdomen, hip, and back all work together to keep the lower back erect and balanced. If any of these muscles is weak, a muscular imbalance can result, causing spinal instability and ultimately back pain and associated problems. Abdominal and back muscles must be balanced and strong for good spinal health. Muscle balance is important throughout the body.

The exercises described in this section are engineered to strengthen the muscles that support your back. They are not designed to increase your muscle mass.

TIPS FOR STRENGTHENING EXERCISES

- Always warm up before the strengthening exercises to increase blood flow, protect joints, and raise muscle temperature. Injury to the muscles, ligaments, and tendons may result if strengthening exercises are begun while the muscles are cold. Mild stretching exercises can help you warm up.
- If an exercise causes pain, cut back on the repetitions, use less force, or stop doing the exercise altogether.
- Remember to breathe normally. Do not hold your breath while exercising. Your tissues need oxygen.

Strengthening Exercise #1: Back Leg Swing (Level 4) This exercise strengthens the hip and back muscles.

- Stand just behind a chair.
- Place your hands on the back of the chair.

- While keeping your right leg straight, lift your left leg back and up as far as possible.
- Hold for 5 seconds.
- Return to the starting position.
- Then keep your left leg straight and lift your right leg back and up as far as possible.
- Hold for 5 seconds.
- Repeat this exercise 5 times.

Strengthening Exercise #2: Leg Side Lift (Level 4) This exercise strengthens the thigh muscles.

- Lie on your left side.
- Tip your pelvis forward.
- Tighten your abdominal muscles.
- Raise your right leg as far as possible (stop if you feel pain in your hip).
- Slightly bend your left knee (about 45 degrees) for better stability.
- Do this exercise 5 or 6 times.
- Repeat the exercise lying on your right side and lifting your left leg.

Strengthening Exercise #3: Bridge the Back (Level 4) This exercise strengthens your buttock, abdominal, and back muscles and improves mobility.

- Lie on your back with your knees bent (about 90 degrees) and your feet flat on the floor a comfortable distance from your hips.
- Your arms should be at your sides.
- Tighten your buttock muscles and lift your pelvis off the floor about 2 to 3 inches.
- Hold for 10 or more seconds.
- Repeat 8 to 10 times.

Strengthening Exercise #4: Mini Sit-Up (Level 4)

This exercise strengthens the abdominal muscles that help support the lower back.

- Lie on the floor with your knees bent at a 90-degree angle. Keep your arms at your sides.

Note: The placement of your hands will influence the difficulty of this exercise.

Easiest: Hands extended straight over the abdomen or at your sides

Harder: Arms crossed over the chest

Hardest: Hands behind the head

- Press the small of your back against the floor.
- Tighten your abdominal muscles and tip your pelvis forward.
- Roll your chin to your chest and slowly raise your head and neck off the floor. Raise up no higher than 30 degrees.
- Continue to tighten abdominal muscles for 5 seconds.
- Slowly relax and return to the floor.
- Repeat 10 times.

Strengthening Exercise #5: Marching on Your Back (Level 4)

This exercise strengthens your abdominal muscles and helps hold your lower back in the proper, pain-free position.

- Lie on your back and put your hands under your hips (keep your lower back on the floor).
- Pull your left knee up to your chest slowly.
- Extend (straighten) the right leg, keeping the leg 6 to 12 inches off the ground.
- Hold about 5 seconds.
- Switch legs, slowly.
- Repeat exercise 8 to 10 times.

Note: If your back begins to hurt before completion, stop.

Strengthening Exercise #6: Hip Hyperextension (Level 5)

This exercise strengthens the muscles of the hips, buttocks, and back.

- Lie on your stomach with your hands and arms extended above your head.
- Straighten your left leg and knee and slowly raise your left leg as high as possible and then lower it 5 times.
- Return to the starting position and relax.
- Straighten and stiffen your right knee and leg and raise and lower it 5 times.
- As you improve in strength, increase until you are doing this exercise 10 times with each leg.

Note: At first, it may be difficult to lift your legs, even slightly, but don't give up. Eventually, you will be able to do it if you keep working at it.

Strengthening Exercise #7: Mule Kicks (Level 4) This exercise strengthens the abdominal muscles.

- Get on your hands and knees. Keep your lower back flat and your lower back and hips even.
- Draw your right knee to your chest and flex your neck (by looking up) and your trunk.
- Then kick your leg back as far as you can, slightly squeezing your buttock muscles while extending your neck and back.
- Raise your leg no higher than parallel to the ground.
- Return to "all fours" position.
- Repeat using your left leg.
- Do 5 times with each leg.

Strengthening Exercise #8: Kicking Up a Storm (Level 4) This exercise improves abdominal strength by improving your pelvic tilt, your endurance, and the balance between the abdomen, pelvis, and back.

- Lie on your back on a bed or platform. The floor or a mat should not be used because, in kicking, the legs go above and below the level of the bed or other surface.

- Extend your feet and legs out from the bed (from the crotch down). Only your hips, torso, head, and arms remain on the bed.
- Tip your pelvis forward and tighten your abdominal muscles, bringing your pelvis closer to your chest plate (sternum).
- With your legs parallel to the ground, begin to alternately raise one leg approximately 12 inches and lower the other 12 inches in a kicking motion.
- Begin slowly and gradually to increase your pace.
- Perform this exercise only as long as you can maintain the pelvic tilt.
- Rest 30 seconds and repeat the exercise.

Note: Initially, perform the exercise no more than 5 times. When the exercise becomes easy to do and your endurance improves, perform the exercise for up to 2 minutes, then relax, then repeat 5 to 10 times, doing this 5 to 7 days a week. For increased resistance (as you progress), wear heavy boots or strap on ankle weights.

Neck-Strengthening Exercises
Isometric (self-resistance) exercises are excellent for strengthening your neck muscles. As your neck strength improves, increase the repetitions and the resistance used to perform the exercise.

Neck-Strengthening Exercise #1: Frontal Resistance (Level 4) This exercise helps strengthen the muscles in the front of your neck.

- Place your palms on your forehead.
- Press your palms against your forehead and resist that action by pushing forward with your head and neck.
- Hold for 5 seconds.
- Slowly relax.
- Repeat this exercise 5 times, twice daily.

Neck-Strengthening Exercise #2: Side Resistance
(Level 4) This exercise strengthens the muscles on the side of the neck.

- Put your right hand against the right side of your head.
- While trying to lower your head to your right shoulder, press your hand against your head, resisting the motion of your head.
- Hold for 5 seconds.
- Relax and repeat on the left side.
- Do this exercise 5 times.

Neck-Strengthening Exercise #3: Back of Neck (Level 4)
This exercise strengthens the muscles in the back of the neck.

- Cup your hands and place them against the back of your head.
- Pushing against your hands, try to push your head backward.
- Hold for 5 seconds.
- Slowly relax.
- Repeat this exercise 5 times.

Neck-Strengthening Exercise #4: Rotational Resistance
(Level 4) This exercise strengthens the muscles of the neck and can improve your range of motion.

- Turn your head as far as you can to the left.
- Place your right hand against the right side of your face.
- While pushing with your hand, try to turn your head back to the right.
- Hold for 5 seconds.
- Slowly relax.
- Repeat this exercise on the opposite side.
- Perform this exercise 5 times on each side.

WEIGHTS AND BODY BUILDING

Some people find it more enjoyable and motivating to exercise and strengthen muscles by using free weights. But be smart when using weights. Many people lift weights only to look good and not to improve their health. "Pooched out" pectorals in the chest, firm gluteal (buttock) muscles, bulging leg quadriceps (on the front of the upper legs), and chiseled abdominal and upper back muscles cause obvious muscle imbalance. In fact, it is not uncommon for weight lifters to have painful lower backs, pulled Achilles tendons, pulled hamstring muscles (in the back of the thighs), or a "hunchback" look because of overdeveloped chest muscles that pull the shoulders abnormally forward.

Of particular concern to me is that more and more children and young adults are acquiring an interest in weight lifting. If your children want to "beef up" in this way, be sure to supervise them carefully. I am reminded of the East Germans in the 1950s and 1960s and the weight-lifting program they developed for young children. As you may know, the East Germans had a massive sports program after World War II. Beginning at ten or eleven years of age, the children were instructed to lift heavy weights. Unfortunately, the children's muscles became overdeveloped, which inhibited normal growth of their bones. The overdeveloped muscles pulled the ends of the long bones of the arms and legs around, giving them a "candle-dripping" appearance—deformed, undersized, and muscle-bound. Needless to say, as soon as they discovered the damage early weight lifting could do, the East Germans drastically changed their training program.

Learn from this example. While your children are still growing, have them do stretching and aerobic exercises. Only when they have stopped growing (at about eighteen to twenty years of age) should children begin lifting weights. A lifetime of pain and discomfort isn't worth being Mr. or Ms. Body Beautiful at sixteen years of age.

AEROBIC TRAINING FOR CARDIOVASCULAR ENDURANCE (LEVELS 4, 5, OR 6, DEPENDING ON THE EXERCISE)

Aerobic exercises bring oxygen to your body's muscles and flame the fires that burn up fat. They help your muscles (including the heart) use oxygen more effectively. With aerobic exercises, you breathe more deeply and pump more oxygenated blood to the various areas of the body. Because painful or fatigued back muscles don't receive enough oxygen, you need aerobic exercises to allow more oxygen-rich blood to reach the back muscles. Further, with aerobic exercises, the body's natural painkilling endorphins are released. Thus, you feel good, have fun, and get on with your life.

Aerobic exercises include running, fast walking, swimming, bicycling (a stationary bike is okay), fast dancing (as opposed to the waltz), jumping rope, and climbing stairs. Be careful of this one. Stop if you experience any pains in the chest. Have fun exercising and stay motivated by asking a friend to work out with you. Don't let a bad climate stop you. Use a treadmill when weather doesn't permit outdoor activities.

Remember, stretching to warm your muscles is always important before aerobic activity. It's also important to stretch after your cardiovascular warm-up. Because muscles are warm, stretching after exercise is the ideal time to minimize stiffness, increase flexibility, and promote circulation. This is also a perfect time to include stress management and relaxation exercises.

Aerobic exercises should be performed at least three to four times per week for twenty to thirty minutes each session. The intensity can vary, but try to maintain your personal target heart rate (see page 184). Take your pulse for six seconds and multiply by ten. If your pulse exceeds your target heart rate, cut back on your intensity. If it is too slow, increase your pace.

Every week or two, complete the Progress Analysis form and the Personal Progress Questionnaire to evaluate your improvement. Be sure to enter the date on each form. As time passes, evaluate your progress, noting changes in your symptoms. This will help you to more accurately judge your actual rate of progress.

PROGRESS ANALYSIS

DATE_____

Important Symptoms (from original case history and questionnaires)

1. _____ Same _____ Better _____ Worse _____
2. _____ Same _____ Better _____ Worse _____
3. _____ Same _____ Better _____ Worse _____
4. _____ Same _____ Better _____ Worse _____
5. _____ Same _____ Better _____ Worse _____
6. _____ Same _____ Better _____ Worse _____

Are there any new symptoms?_____

How would you evaluate your progress in general?_____

PERSONAL PROGRESS QUESTIONNAIRE

Answer all questions that apply.

Today's date _____
Date you first felt your back pain _____
Date you began the Five-Step Jump-Start Plus Program

_____

1. What questions do you have about your condition or progress to date?

_____
_____
_____
_____
_____
_____
_____
_____

2. What symptoms have improved?

_____

_____

_____

_____

_____

_____

_____

3. Changes in general. Are you:

Stronger?	YES	NO
More alert?	YES	NO
More relaxed?	YES	NO
More restful	YES	NO

4. Activities that are easier to do:

Walking	YES	NO
Working	YES	NO
Sitting	YES	NO
Standing	YES	NO
Lifting	YES	NO
Bending	YES	NO
Riding	YES	NO
Sleeping	YES	NO

5. Conditions that have improved:

Nerve reflexes	YES	NO
Digestion	YES	NO
Elimination	YES	NO
Pain	YES	NO
Muscle strength	YES	NO
Headaches	YES	NO
Breathing	YES	NO
Back or neck ache	YES	NO

6. Are you improving?_____

7. Are there any new symptoms? YES NO
   If so, list them. _____

8. On a scale of 0 to 10, where 0 is no pain and 10 is
   extreme pain, indicate your present level of pain:

Head and neck

| | | | | | | | | | | |
0 1 2 3 4 5 6 7 8 9 10

Thoracic region (mid back)

| | | | | | | | | | | |
0 1 2 3 4 5 6 7 8 9 10

Lumbar region (lower back)

| | | | | | | | | | | |
0 1 2 3 4 5 6 7 8 9 10

Review your completed form and compare it with any previous
forms to help you evaluate your progress. If you have a new injury,
complete a new form. This information will give you a record of your
back pain and the most successful ways to care for your own back.

HOW TO FIGURE YOUR TARGET HEART RATE
It only takes a few seconds to find your target heart rate
using this formula.

Start with the number 220:   220

Then subtract your age: − ____

Subtotal: ____

This number is your "predicted maximum heart rate,"
or the maximum pulse for your age. From this number,
subtract your resting heart rate (the number of times
your heart beats per minute when you are at rest):   − ____

Subtotal: _____

Multiply the subtotal by 50 to 85 percent, depending on your activity and fitness level. A beginning exerciser should use 50 percent, an intermediate exerciser 70 percent, and a competitive athlete 85 percent.   x _____

Subtotal: _____

To this number, add your resting heart rate (from above): + _____

This is your target heart rate—the rate you should try to maintain during aerobic exercise: _____

For instance, a thirty-year-old woman just beginning to exercise would compute her target heart rate as follows:

Beginning number:	220
Subtract her age:	– 30
Predicted maximum heart rate:	190
Subtract her resting heart rate (72):	– 72
	118

Because our thirty-year-old is a beginner, she'll multiply by 50 percent, or 0.50:	x Ø.50
	59
Add her resting heart rate:	+ 72
Our beginning exerciser's target heart rate:	131

YOGA

For over five thousand years, yoga has been used to attain superior health and flexibility, maintain vitality, and reduce stress. Yoga is a method to improve health and beat back pain through meditation, stretching, breathing, relaxation, and exercise.

Yoga is simple and easy to perform. Very popular in India and many other countries, yoga only became popular in the United States during the 1960s through the work of B. K. S. Iyengar and Swami Vishnudevananda and their illustrated yoga manuals.

Yoga can bring a brief peaceful interlude to your hectic daily life, enabling you to relax. Yoga can invigorate your body and your mind and allow you to face life with more positive awareness. Yoga helps you to "walk in balance."

The number of yoga postures is voluminous. According to Eleanor Criswell, author of *How Yoga Works: An Introduction to Somatic Yoga*, there are some eighty-four thousand variations.[2] Although yoga exercises lead to the same goal, their movements vary.

The following basic yoga exercises have been chosen to help you gain improved overall mobility and healing. If a posture causes pain, don't do it. Yoga should only be performed by those in good health. Those with severe back pain should not attempt yoga until their condition has improved and they have received approval from their physician. In addition, pregnant women should consult with their physician before beginning any exercise or yoga program.

Begin with a basic set of postures, which could include the corpse, the fish, the cobra, and the half locust. The key is to do what you can. Remember: If any exercise causes back pain, don't do it. As your back and flexibility improve, you can add additional postures, with caution. Consult any reference book on yoga for additional exercises.

The Corpse (Level 1) The corpse pose is one of the easiest yoga positions to learn and practice. With this position, the mind and body are relaxed, and nerves and muscles are restored, soothed, and rested. Some feel that this position removes the biochemical effects of fatigue, helps the venous blood return to the heart more easily, and decreases blood pressure.

- The initial position is to lie on the floor on your back with your legs stretched out. Place your feet about 20 inches apart.
- Place your arms at your sides, with your hands approximately 10 inches away from your body with the palms up.
- Make your body and back as balanced and relaxed as possible. Do not unconsciously arch your back. To make

sure you are relaxed, roll your head slightly and move your feet.

■ Breathe deeply when doing the corpse position. Abdominal deep breathing for 1 minute is suggested to supply the body with increased oxygen. This encourages relaxation and helps you to practice visualization. Count to 4 while inhaling and count to 4 while exhaling 8 times. Each count should be about 1 second. Be sure to breathe in and out easily and quietly. There should be no effort involved.

The Fish (Level 2) This position helps facilitate good posture and brings fresh input to your nervous system. The fish posture seems to help the back, neck, and chest muscles. The flexor muscles of the chest are relaxed, while the trapezius muscles are contracted. This helps the back become more relaxed and more comfortable by releasing muscle tension.

■ To begin the fish, sit on the floor with your legs flat and stretched out in front of you.
■ Gently place your elbows on the floor behind you.
■ Ease your head behind you down to the floor (the neck is bent back in this position).
■ In that position, slowly look toward the floor behind you, bending your neck.
■ Relax and hold that position for 20 counts.
■ Each time you repeat this yoga exercise, extend the time by about 30 counts.
■ The maximum time recommended for this position is no more than 3 minutes.
■ When you have assumed this position, remember to relax the entire body and breathe normally.
■ Remember all the sensations of this posture to help improve posture and nervous system function.

The Cobra (Level 1) By contracting and relaxing back muscles, the cobra position helps strengthen the back (particularly the extensor muscles of the lower back) while simultaneously relaxing the muscles of the abdomen. In certain conditions, the cobra position can help reposition spinal vertebral displacements. The cobra pose apparently stimulates the nervous system, which has its pathway along the spinal column.

- Begin by lying facedown on the floor with your legs stretched out and your feet together.
- Place your palms on the floor beside your shoulders.
- Inhale deeply.
- Gradually elevate your chest off the ground. You should feel each vertebra lift.
- Visualize that as you inhale, you are being lifted from the ground.
- Keep your eyes open and look toward the ceiling.
- Hold this position and count to 10.
- Relax and slowly exhale.
- Inhale and repeat the movement 3 times.
- End the cobra pose with some movement or posture that relaxes the lower back and contracts the abdominal muscles. This is to relieve tightness in your lower back and to keep you from hyperextending your back.

The Half Locust (Level 1) The locust pose helps improve circulation to the legs and tones abdominal muscles. Toning abdominal muscles can help flatten the back, thus decreasing the lower back curve and taking pressure off your lower back.

- Begin by lying facedown on your stomach with your head resting on your chin.
- Place your arms at your sides and your palms on the floor.
- Inhale while extending one leg in the air as much as possible. Hold the position for 10 counts.
- Slowly lower the leg while exhaling.
- Repeat the process with the other leg.
- Repeat the half locust posture 3 to 7 times for each leg.
- Holding the posture for extended time periods can lead to calmness and relaxation.

As your back pain decreases, use regular, intelligent stretching as an integral part of yoga. This allows people of all ages to remain flexible and pain free. Additional yoga stretches found in the May/June 1996 issue of *Yoga Journal* ("The Ten Most Important Stretches," by Judith Lasater) augment my program of beating back pain.[3] These exercises are good for stretching the hamstring muscles, calf muscles, front thigh (quadricep) muscles, inner thigh muscles, shoulder muscles, biceps, triceps, midback muscles, hip rotator muscles, and muscles of the lower back. The majority of these exercises are a level 3 on my difficulty scale.

According to John Abbott, publisher of *Yoga Journal*, individuals should attend yoga classes and practice yoga under the direction of a yoga master. Working with others gives positive reinforcement. Therefore, use this book, videotapes, and classes for permanent success and increased harmony. If Vanda Scaravelli, a powerful, slight woman in her mid-eighties ("Awakening the Spine" by Esther Myers and Kim Echlin, *Yoga Journal*, May/June 1996, 66–73)[4] can do yoga, so can you.

QI GONG (OR CHI KUNG OR CH'I KUNG)

The ancient meditative exercise called qi gong is an excellent way to relax, meditate, and perform physical exercise. Qi gong is a traditional Chinese form of exercise for healing the mind, body, and spirit and finding inner harmony, strength, optimal health, and peace. Chinese masters, thousands of years ago, developed a series of gentle movements that channel qi (often spelled *chi*—the life force) into the body for energizing, healing, and detoxifying. Through qi gong, you learn to build a reserve of energy, quickly increase vitality with a few self-massage techniques, and "vibrate" inner toxins away from the body. Qi gong can be integrated into the Five-Step Jump-Start Plus Program.

By adjusting and improving your body posture, mental capacity, breathing cycle, and nervous system, qi gong helps to improve internal function, to correct or restore health, and to resist many chronic disorders, including back problems, arthritis, hypertension, anxiety, and coronary heart disease.

The following qi gong exercises are designed to help relieve back pain and joint pain. Daily practice is important to help you learn the various techniques. As with any exercise, if you feel any pain, stop immediately. Qi gong is a continuous, flowing exercise, but some of the motions may be difficult for you to perform.

In the qi gong exercises described here, begin by standing naturally with your whole body relaxed. If you cannot stand, there are also qi gong exercises performed from a sitting position. Please see one of the many books available on qi gong for additional exercises.

First Exercise (Level 3)

- Stand in a relaxed position with your legs slightly bent at the knees.
- Move your arms in a circular fashion backward and up.
- Spread your chest.
- Bring your shoulders back.
- Breathe in deeply.
- Bend your head forward but not lower than the waist.
- Remain in this position for 6 rotations of your arms.
- Return to a relaxed standing position.
- Relax your chest and shoulders.
- Breathe deeply.

Note: If you feel dizzy at any time during this exercise, return to your relaxed upright position immediately.

Second Exercise (Level 3)

- Stand in a relaxed position with your legs slightly bent at the knees.
- Place your hands above your hips toward the back (over the kidneys).
- Rotate the upper body from the hips and the waist in a clockwise direction.
- Make 6 full circles of rotation.
- After this, rotate from the hips and waist in a counterclockwise direction.

- Make 6 full circles of rotation.
- Breathe naturally in and out during this exercise.

Third Exercise (Level 3)
- Stand in a relaxed position with your legs slightly bent at the knees. Your feet should be shoulder-width apart and should not move during this exercise.
- Take a deep breath.
- Bend forward as far as possible. Let your hands hang relaxed and down.
- Exhale deeply as you bend over.
- Now breathe easily and naturally.
- Begin making a very large imaginary circle by swinging both arms slowly to the right. Your left hand should cross in front of your legs.
- As your hands move up, your body should move up with them and straighten.
- As your arms reach over your head, your palms should now be turned forward.
- Your arms and hands should pass over your head and begin to descend on your left side.
- As the hands descend and reach the waist, begin to bend forward from the waist.
- The legs should be relaxed, slightly bent at the knees but relatively straight.
- Return to the initial exercise position. That is, your back should be bent forward as far as possible and your arms and hands should be hanging down in a relaxed position.
- This exercise should be one of continual motion. Therefore, after completing one circle, continue immediately into a second and third circle.
- After completing 3 circles in one direction, repeat in the opposite direction.
- When the 3 circles are completed in both directions, slowly return to your relaxed, upright, standing position.
- As you return, think of each vertebra in your back as a separate entity. As you straighten up, visualize that you are like a brick layer, placing one vertebra on top of the next, keeping each in alignment.

- As you come to an upright position, pull in your abdominal muscles, tip your pelvis forward, extend your chest, roll your shoulders back, and bring your head to a comfortably balanced position on the top of the spine, with your chin tucked in and your eyes looking forward.
- Inhale deeply, then exhale deeply, conceptualizing that all the stress and blocks of vital energy are leaving your body.

Fourth Exercise (Level 3)
- Stand in a relaxed position.
- Raise your arms shoulder height.
- Breathe in deeply.
- Lower your hands slowly until they reach waist level.
- Simultaneously, bend your knees.
- Breathe out deeply.
- Then raise your arms.
- Straighten your legs.
- Breathe in deeply.
- Breathe out deeply.
- Perform 10 times.

Fifth Exercise (Level 3)
- Stand in a relaxed position.
- Raise your shoulders.
- Bring your shoulders back and spread your chest.
- Breathe in deeply.
- Roll your shoulders forward, down, and in.
- Draw in your chest.
- Bend your neck and back slightly forward.
- Bend your knees.
- Exhale deeply.
- Perform 10 times.

Sixth Exercise (Level 3)
- Stand in a relaxed position.
- Lift your legs up and down as you march in place.
- Lift your knees so that your thighs are parallel to the ground.

- Gently swing your hands and arms forward and backward.
- Your shoulders should be level.
- Start with homolateral movement—that is, move the same foot and hand forward, such as the right foot and right hand moving together, then the left foot and left hand.
- After 5 or 6 repetitions of homolateral movement, switch to contralateral movement—that is, swinging the right arm forward and simultaneously bringing the left leg up, then the left arm and the right leg, and so on. Make the movements relaxed, smooth, and easy.
- Do 10 repetitions of marching with opposite arms and legs.

Note: This exercise is similar to cross-patterning, only you are not walking but marching in place.

TAI CHI

Tai chi chuan is a form of movement developed thousands of years ago from the martial arts in China. Commonly referred to as tai chi, this traditional Chinese form of exercise combines relaxation and deep diaphragmatic breathing with gentle and slow movements.

Although there are various schools of tai chi chuan, three essential features are always emphasized:

1. The mind is tranquil but alert, with a strong body-mind relationship and with consciousness commanding the body.
2. The body is naturally relaxed and extended.
3. Body movements are well coordinated, slow, and smooth throughout the entire exercise period. Movements should flow from one to another effortlessly—that is, without expenditures of excess energy from unnecessary contraction of muscles.

Scientific studies of tai chi chuan have shown its value in improving balance, postural control, and movement. Professor Bert H. Jacobson and associates of the School of

Health, Physical Education and Leisure, Oklahoma State University, compared two groups of twelve volunteers ranging in age from twenty to forty-five years.[5] One group used tai chi training for twelve weeks; the other group did not. Those who practiced tai chi had better lateral body stability, balance, and strength of maximal knee extension, as well as better body balance. Jacobson and his colleagues feel that when individuals have balance and postural control, they maintain equilibrium in their bodies and can better control their movements.

The benefits of tai chi on older adults was studied by Professor Nancy G. Kutner and associates of the Department of Rehabilitation Medicine, School of Medicine, Emory University, in Atlanta, Georgia.[6] One hundred and thirty subjects over seventy years of age were randomly placed in a tai chi exercise program for fifteen weeks. Follow-up assessments revealed that the adults who had participated in tai chi were significantly more likely to report a positive effect on their lives and on activities of daily life. There was a change in their normal physical activity, and they felt that they had benefited from their tai chi chuan, had developed increased body awareness, and had redirected their stress. They felt more energy and strength, improved "focus" and concentration, a sense of achievement and confidence, and better coordination and balance.

How does tai chi compare with exercises such as swimming or jogging? Individuals who regularly practiced tai chi for a number of years feel that they can work for longer periods of time or climb stairs without experiencing fatigue, according to Herman Kauz in *Tai Chi Handbook*.[7] With tai chi, there are no extreme or quick movements. Thus, there seems no possibility of pulled or torn muscles. Regular tai chi has been shown to improve muscle strength, flexibility, and balance as well as circulation and immune function.

Tai Chi Exercises

Don't forget to breathe during the entire tai chi series of movements. For each movement, take a deep inhalation through your nose and then exhale completely through your mouth. This facilitates the flow of chi. Focus your controlled breathing, and concentrate your inner energy.

Focus your mental energy flowing into the body part involved in the movement. Keep your mind relaxed and in a peaceful state. Eliminate all excitement and distractions. It's important to concentrate while doing the movements.

Warm-Up Exercises (All Level 3) As with any exercise, please be sure to loosen up first. The following are simple warm-up exercises. Be sure to make all movements continuous, slow, and without stress. If you are limited in your movements because of back pain or physical restrictions, only do what you can. Don't force it.

1. Loosen Your Ankle Joints
   - Stand with your feet shoulder-width apart.
   - Put your weight on your left foot.
   - Slide your right foot back about 1 to 2 feet.
   - Keeping the ball of the right foot on the floor, rotate the ankle 5 times to the right, then 5 times to the left.
   - Step up with your right foot.
   - Slide the left foot back and repeat the process.
   - Be sure to make all movements slowly, evenly, and continuously.

2. Loosen Your Knees
   - Stand in an upright position.
   - Bend your knees slightly (about 15 to 30 degrees). Bend your knees only as low as is comfortable. Don't go down too low.
   - Put your hands on your knees.
   - Move your knees in a circular fashion 5 times in one direction, then 5 times in the other direction.
   - Move your knees slowly, easily, and continuously.

3. Bend and Touch Exercise
   - Stand with your feet about two shoulder-widths apart.

- Extend your arms out from your shoulders at shoulder height.
- Be sure to bend your knees with each exercise.
- With the right hand, reach over and touch the floor in front of your left foot.
- Then return to the upright position.
- Repeat with the left hand and right foot.
- Repeat the sequence 5 times.

4. Hip Rotation
   - Stand with your feet shoulder-width apart.
   - Place your hands on your hips.
   - Turn your hips in full circles, first one way and then the other—5 times one way, and then 5 times the other.
   - Make the movements a slow, continuous, and smooth rotation of the hips.
   - Work within your capacity.

5. Waist Rotation
   - Raise your arms in front of your chest. Your hands should be lightly clenched.
   - Stand with your feet shoulder-width apart.
   - Relax your shoulders.
   - From the waist, turn your upper body from side to side 5 times.
   - Don't overstretch.
   - Make sure your movements are smooth and continuous.

6. Side-Bending Exercise
   - Stand comfortably with your feet shoulder-width apart.
   - Raise your right hand over your head.
   - Keep all movements slow, smooth, and continuous.
   - Slowly drop your right arm to your side.

- Repeat the process with your left hand.
- Repeat the exercise 5 times.
- Don't overdo it.

7. Shoulder Roll
   - Stand comfortably with your feet shoulder-width apart.
   - Let your arms hang loosely at your sides.
   - Roll both your shoulders, moving them up, back, down, then up and back to the starting position. Make the circle as wide as possible.
   - Repeat 5 times.
   - Then roll your shoulders in the opposite direction— forward, down, then up and back to neutral.
   - Repeat 5 times.

Note: You can alternately roll one shoulder and then the other.

8. Upper Back Stretch
   - Stand comfortably with your feet together.
   - Move your toes out 45 degrees with heels together.
   - Relax your body.
   - Let your arms hang loosely at your sides.
   - Reach back with your hands and clasp them behind your back (palms together and fingers interlaced).
   - Stretch your neck up.
   - Roll your shoulders forward.
   - Attempt to bring your elbows together as close as possible.
   - Hold for 5 to 10 seconds.
   - Relax your shoulders and arms.
   - Roll your shoulders forward to beginning stance.
   - Repeat upper back stretch 5 times.

Now that you are warmed up, try the following tai chi exercises. But first assume the beginning position.

Beginning Position (Level 4)

- Hold your head in a naturally straight and upright position.
- The tip of your tongue should touch the upper palate. Your upper teeth should gently touch your lower teeth. Don't clench your teeth.
- Keep your neck relaxed and upright.
- Your shoulders and arms should hang down naturally and relaxed.
- Keep your spine straight and relaxed.
- Keep the buttocks relaxed and tucked in slightly.
- Look straight ahead; then, during the exercise as you move your arms or hands, monitor them with your eyes.
- Any arm movement should be circular and with an even flow, allowing the energy to pass through your arms.
- Make all movements slow, continuous, and even.

First Exercise (Yu Bei Shi) (Level 4)

- Stand with your weight balanced evenly on both legs.
- Your toes should be pointing straight ahead.
- Shift your weight completely onto the right foot.
- Raise your left foot, move it about shoulder-width apart from the right foot, and shift all of your weight to the left foot.
- With the palms facing backward, lift and bend your elbows to the side.
- Now place equal weight on both feet.
- Slump your shoulders by bringing them forward. This will also depress your chest.
- Your back should be as straight as possible, and the body should be completely relaxed.
- This exercise allows chi to sink to the Dantian—the center of all energy in your body (deep in the body and about three fingers down from your bellybutton).
- Focus your energy on the Dantian. Store energy (chi).
- Inhale deeply, then exhale deeply.
- Look straight ahead.

Second Exercise (Qi Shi) (Level 4)

- Gradually raise your arms upward and forward to shoulder height.
- Keep your palms down and relax the fingers.
- Extend your fingers slowly until they point forward.
- Focus on the Dantian.
- Inhale deeply.
- Look straight ahead.
- Gradually bend your elbows and move your hands back toward your chest.
- Slightly lower both elbows.
- Move your fingers upward slightly.
- Then lower your hands slowly to just below the hips.
- Palms should face the body.
- Slightly bend the elbows outward.
- Allow your fingers to hang down slightly.
- Focus on the Dantian.
- Exhale deeply.
- Look straight ahead.

Tae-Bo

Personally developed by seven-time world martial arts champion Billy Blanks, tae-bo is a combination of stretching exercises, plus dance, boxing, and the ancient arts of self-defense. *Tae* is from the Korean word for "foot," and *bo* is for "boxing." The tae-bo style of aerobic kickboxing is reported to burn up to 800 calories per hour. Many movie stars and professional athletes use this exercise technique. Because this program works every body part, it aids in strengthening and toning muscles as well as in losing weight.

For more information on tae-bo, contact Tae-Bo, 7095 Hollywood Boulevard, Hollywood, CA 90028 (telephone: [877] 228-2326).

ADDITIONAL TRADITIONAL CHINESE MEDICINE AND HOLISTIC THERAPIES FOR BACK PAIN

In addition to exercise, many manual techniques and physical rehabilitation modalities can be helpful in relieving your back problem. These can include everything from chiropractic adjustments to massage. The following techniques, modalities, and orthotics are all things you can do to help relieve back pain.

Acupressure

Acupressure uses the same principles as acupuncture but with pressure rather than needles. The technique originated in China and Japan over three thousand years ago and is a combination of acupuncture and massage.

Clinically, acupressure has been shown to help fight backache, "slipped disk," strains and sprains, sciatica, and general pain, and it is very effective in relieving certain types of back pain.

You can apply acupressure by yourself, but if you are unable to reach certain acupoints to relieve your pain, get a partner to help.

Acupressure for Backache

- Be sure you are not disturbed. Disconnect your telephone if necessary.
- Try to maintain a relaxing, calm, and quiet environment. Playing low-key, relaxing background music may be helpful.
- Sit in a chair or on the floor or lie down on a bed.
- Do not drink alcoholic beverages or take any painkillers or any other medication before treatment.
- Find the correct acupressure point. Gently touch your skin around the area where the point should be located. Check to see if one point is more sensitive than another. Then mark the point(s) with a felt-tip pen for easy reference.
- In back pain, the correct acupressure points are often located near the sacrum and between the coccyx and the sacrum. If this is true in your case, using your thumb,

index finger, or middle finger, press in the hollow of the sacrum and also between the coccyx and the sacrum. Press for 3 to 5 seconds.

- While pressing, exercise breath control (breathe from the diaphragm).
- Do this 5 to 10 times in a row but for no more than 25 minutes of treatment.
- Make sure you have plenty of time to relax and concentrate on what you are doing.
- Stop immediately if you feel pain.
- Treat acute conditions (pain) 3 times per day and chronic conditions (pain) once per day (no more than 25 minutes).
- For acupressure points on your back or other places inaccessible for self-treatment, ask a partner for help.

Remember, acupressure cannot substitute if surgery is required. See a trained acupuncturist or physician if you have questions. *Note:* You should not use acupressure if you have a serious inflammatory, circulatory, or cardiac disorder or a skin condition (especially with a pus discharge).

See Suggested Reading and Viewing for a list of helpful books on acupressure.

Aromatherapy

Aromatherapy—the art of using essential oils for health and beauty—is several centuries old and is an excellent aid to relaxation. Aromatherapy is a healing system used as a complement to other therapies, such as acupressure, pressure-point therapy, and massage. We know that the ancient Egyptians used scented ointments and that the Greeks and Romans employed essential oils during massage and steam baths. If your mother put menthol in a vaporizer to ease your breathing when you were a child, she was using aromatherapy.

Essential oils (highly concentrated extracts from plants) can be inhaled, applied directly to the skin through massage, used in a compress, or applied indirectly (for example, when used in bathwater). Table 9.2 lists a number of oils for specific back conditions.

According to aromatherapy researcher Alexandra Avery,

author of *Aromatherapy and You: A Guide to Natural Skin Care,* "The sense of smell is the most expedient and direct connection to the brain of all the five senses."[8] In fact, she notes that our sense of smell is ten thousand times more sensitive than our sense of taste and that our olfactory system may even contain more receptor cells than the eyes. Avery maintains that there is a physiological response when inhaling the aroma of a flower or of an essential oil.

To relieve anxiety and nervous tension, try the following essential oils, available at health food stores and many department stores:

bergamot	myrrh
geranium	neroli
jasmine	rose
lavender	ylang-ylang
marjoram	

Table 9.2

AROMATIC OILS FOR VARIOUS BACK CONDITIONS

CONDITION	AROMATIC OIL
Arthritis	Juniper, eucalyptus
Backache	Sandalwood
Joint pains	Juniper, eucalyptus
Lumbago	Rosemary, tea tree
Rheumatism	Chamomile, tea tree, sage oil
Sciatica	Chamomile, sandalwood
Slipped disk	Rosemary

Note: Experts do not recommend the ingestion or internal use of essential oils. These are highly concentrated, powerful essences, and any internal use should only be at the direction, and under the close supervision, of a trained health care practitioner.

Back Braces, Corsets, and Other Supports

A back brace, corset, or other support can help compress the abdominal muscles and lend support to the lower back. Such devices may also help control pain and prevent injury because they limit bending.

These supports are available in many drugstores and from your physician. They are made from a variety of materials, including canvas, elastic, neoprene, rigid plastic, and metal. Some close with Velcro, while others may have snaps, buckles, belts, zippers, or other closures. Some have shoulder straps for additional support, while others have a hard plastic or Styrofoam insert that slips into a pocket in the back for extra strength.

For best results, a brace, corset, or other back support should fit like work gloves—that is, snug without being restrictive. It should be worn when extra back protection is required, such as when there are unavoidable work or household tasks involving lifting or bending, or when you must sit for long periods, such as while at work or while traveling.

Balm

A balm is an aromatic ointment with soothing and healing properties. Balms are frequently used in massage therapy as topical analgesics. Commercial balms such as Thera-Gesic from Mission Pharmacal Company often contain methyl salicylate and menthol, but you can also make your own balm to relax muscles, decrease stress, and decrease many inflammations of the skin.

Lemon Balm

■ Mix lemon balm oil (3 to 5 drops) with $1^{1}/_{2}$ ounces of a base oil (such as wheat germ oil, sweet almond oil, or olive oil).

■ Store in a sealed container.

■ To use, massage the balm on the back and into the tissues on either side of the spine.

Baths

Baths can help increase overall body circulation, bring nutrients to the tissues, and remove toxins, especially on the skin and near the skin's surface. Baths can also improve absorption of nutrients through the skin and remove dead superficial tissue.

Treating physical ills by immersion in water, such as in heated pools, whirlpools, or Hubbard tanks (stainless steel tanks of heated, circulating water), is called *hydrotherapy*. Heat can relax the muscles and reduce muscle spasms, increase the flexibility of muscles, tendons, and ligaments, and relieve pain. It also increases blood flow to the target area and thereby accelerates healing.

A Jacuzzi or hot tub can be relaxing and help soothe back muscles. However, if you are experiencing back pain, care must be taken to avoid reinjuring your back while getting in and out of the tub.

Hot herbal baths using chamomile, hops, or valerian can be very relaxing. A wonderful technique is to put the herbs in a handkerchief or large cloth bag. Tie the bag to the tub's faucet. For a few minutes, let hot water run from the faucet through the bag. Then adjust the water temperature to a comfortable level.

Baths for Back Pain Relief

- Soak comfortably in hot bathwater to which you have added leaves or buds of birch and/or some eucalyptus oil or essence.
- Take seaweed baths daily. Add a handful of seaweed to warm water. The water should be as warm as possible for the elements from the seaweed to be absorbed into the skin. The body's metabolism can be stimulated as the heat penetrates into the body from the dilated skin surface.
- Mugwort baths are frequently used in TCM for rheumatism and nerve pain and to improve circulation and relieve back pain.
  - Add two to three handfuls of dried mugwort leaves to 1 to 2 quarts of water.

- Bring the water to a boil.
- After the water comes to a boil, strain the leaves and add the remaining liquid to the bathwater.
- Check the temperature of the water before entering the bath.

Cervical Collars

Immediately after an injury such as whiplash, it may be beneficial to wear a cervical collar to support the head. A cervical collar is a support, often made of firm foam rubber with a Velcro fastener. The support wraps around the neck and helps hold the head in an upright position. This helps reduce the pressure on the damaged neck muscles and ligaments.

Cervical Pillows

A healthy neck (called the cervical region) has a forward curve much like the letter *c*. Significant neck pain can occur if muscular weakness due to injury or degeneration causes the neck's curve to be diminished or if the neck curves in the wrong direction (backward rather than forward). Lying on a cervical pillow can help support the neck and help return its normal C-shaped curve. A cervical pillow is a pillow formed in such a way as to give extra support to the neck and help maintain its natural curvature. Cervical pillows are usually made from polyurethane foam or fiberfill.

Compresses

A compress is a pad of cloth, gauze, or other material applied with pressure that may be heated or used cold and that may be dry or wet if soaked in an herbal infusion or other liquid or medication. The purpose of a warm compress is to dilate blood vessels, thus increasing circulation. A cold compress can constrict blood vessels, thus decreasing swelling and pain. The following compresses are recommended for sore or strained muscles and sprained ligaments.

Sugar/Onion Compress

- Prepare a compress by mixing $1/2$ cup of granulated sugar and 2 tablespoons of grated onion in 1 cup of warm water.

- Soak a cloth or gauze in the mixture, and then wring out any excess liquid.
- Apply the compress to the problem area and keep in place until the compress begins to cool.
- This compress seems to soothe pulled ligaments and muscles. Change at least three times per day.

Hot Milk Compress
- Prepare a compress of hot fresh milk.
- Apply to the problem area.
- Change at least three times per day.

Heat
Heat is one of the oldest modalities for pain relief. Heat can also improve function and relax the muscles, decreasing muscle spasms. Sources of superficial heat include hot-water bottles, hot packs, hot moist compresses, gel or chemical packs, electric heating pads, and Thermaphor moisture-attracting electric warmer pads (available at drugstores). Chiropractors, naturopaths, and physical therapists may also use a hydrocollator heat-retaining pad or deep heating, which creates heat from energy. Diathermy (shortwave, microwave) and ultrasound therapy are other examples of deep heating.

Superficial heat raises tissue temperature in the body, dilating the superficial blood vessels and thus helping to bring oxygenated blood to the damaged area, which speeds healing. While warm applications can be helpful for moderate pain by relaxing and soothing muscle spasms, cold is generally more effective in decreasing or alleviating musculoskeletal pain.

Note: A heating pad should never be used for more than twenty minutes in any one-hour period. Be careful never to fall asleep while using a heating pad on your body. Who wants both back pain and a burn?

Heel Lifts
Heel lifts (insoles) are devices placed inside shoes that can help equalize uneven leg length. This, in turn, can help reduce back pain. A study on patients with mild back pain

found that 44 percent experienced a reduction in back pain when using shoe insoles.[9]

Available as inexpensive over-the-counter inserts (made from rubber or foam), heel lifts can also be custom-made based on precise foot measurements and impressions taken by your physician.

Ice Massage and Ice Packs

Cold is a very effective pain reliever. It helps decrease pain by numbing the nerves that transmit painful messages. Ice also decreases the size of small blood vessels (capillaries and arterioles). This limits the rate at which fluid escapes into the damaged area, thus decreasing swelling, pain, and inflammation and giving the body time to remove waste products from the damaged area and allow nutrients into the damaged area. Ice massage should be used immediately after any acute injury and can be an effective pain reliever when applied over painful areas for one to five minutes every hour. This should be done a minimum of three to four times a day over very tender spots and trigger points (or pressure points). (See "Trigger-Point Therapy," page 217).

You can make an ice applicator by freezing a popsicle stick or a tongue depressor in a paper cup of water. The stick will act like a handle and can improve your reach. It also makes the frozen cup easier to hold. When ready to use the ice, tear off the top 1/4 inch of the paper. Gently massage the affected area with firm strokes until the area is numb. It is important to keep moving the ice in a circular fashion and never let it rest in one place on the skin. First you will feel the skin begin to cool, then you will feel a burning sensation for a few minutes, and finally you will feel numbness and pain relief. Continue about one minute after the numbness has been experienced. Stop if the area begins to hurt. *Note:* Prolonged application of ice can cause frostbite. Ice is a great therapy, but caution is warranted.

Commercially prepared chemical cold packs or gel packs can also be used and are readily available at drugstores and grocery stores. Wrap the cold pack in a dish towel before applying to the skin. Apply cold packs fifteen minutes on and fifteen minutes off. They are helpful and safe in relieving pain.

Liniments
A liniment can be a paste or liquid and is frequently oil based. Liniments are rubbed and massaged into the skin. Depending on its contents, a liniment can be effective as a local anesthetic, as a lubricant for its soothing effects, as a skin warmer, or as a soothing counterirritant. Liniments are used to treat aching joints (such as arthritis) and muscles, strains and sprains, back pain, and rheumatism. Effective liniments can be made from the oils of marigold, garlic, chiles, and almonds. Because methyl salicylate can be absorbed through the skin, it is the most common commercial ingredient. Do not use a heating pad with liniments because this process can cause blisters. (Also see "Paste," page 215.)

Liniment for an Aching Back
For back, joint, and rheumatic pain, TCM notes this liniment:

1. Combine 1 cup of very good olive oil with $1/2$ cup of lanolin.
2. Place in a glass or mason jar.
3. Allow to stand for twenty-four hours.
4. Place 1 tablespoon of liniment into your hand and massage into aching areas of the back.
5. Cover with gauze or cloth, wrapping the material around the torso.
6. Change the cloth two to three times per day until back pain subsides.

Magnetic Field Therapy
The human body produces subtle magnetic fields. Generated by nervous system ionic currents or by chemical reactions within the cells, these fields can be disturbed by illness and injury. Enzymes, the catalysts responsible for all activity in the human body, help produce magnetic fields, are driven by magnetic fields, and can be affected by magnetic fields.

In recent years, scientists have found that the body's

functions can be affected negatively and positively by external magnetic fields. Magnetic therapy promotes recovery by restoring the body's own normal magnetic field to a healthy state.

Research shows that magnetic therapy is effective in treating such conditions as arthritis, neck and back injuries, sciatic pain, sports injuries, intervertebral disk problems, and even cancer and other degenerative disorders. Magnetic field therapy can fight the effects of stress, facilitate the repair of broken bones, and eliminate pain (including back pain).

Magnets have two poles, negative and positive. The brain registers pain both locally and generally throughout the body as a positive magnetic field. Therefore, by exposing the body to a negative magnetic field, you can return the body's balance and relieve pain. It is generally agreed that the positive pole has a stressful effect, while the negative pole helps normalize metabolic function and has a calming effect.

In treating back pain, place a suitably sized magnet (negative side facing the body) over the painful area. Because the opposite pole surrounds the edge of a magnet, the magnet must extend over the site, that is, the site must be smaller than the magnet. Pain relief may occur within ten to fifteen minutes, but you may require a longer period.

A magnet's strength is measured in gauss units or in teslas (1 tesla equals 10,000 gauss). A manufacturer's gauss rating should accompany any magnetic device or magnet. Remember, the strength of a magnet quickly decreases the farther it is placed from the subject.

Different polarities and different gauss strengths can be used for various therapeutic purposes, according to William H. Philpott, M.D., an internationally known expert on magnets.[10] The more complex or serious the condition, the higher must be the magnetic strength (about 3,500 gauss and up, says Dr. Philpott). However, for lesser conditions, lower-strength magnetic therapy (850 gauss or less) can be effective.

Magnetic products can be purchased through the following companies:

Tools for Exploration
4460 Redwood Highway, Suite 2
San Rafael, CA 94903
Tel: (415) 499-9080 or 1-800-456-9887
Fax: (415) 499-9047

Nikken USA, Inc.
15363 Barranca Parkway
Irvine, CA 92718
Tel: (714) 789-2000
Fax: (714) 789-2080

Massage

Almost everyone feels better after a good massage. Massage is a healing technique used in the East and West alike, though techniques might differ slightly.

Both Chinese and Western massage techniques improve circulation, draw off toxic waste products, relax the muscles, relieve muscle spasms, and decrease muscle stiffness. Massage can stimulate, invigorate, and relax the body and mind, treat heart disorders, improve circulation, reduce hypertension, and relieve depression, tension, hyperactivity, insomnia, sinusitis, and migraine. It can also decrease swelling, pain, and stiffness and is widely used in the treatment of back pain.

Massage is used to treat rheumatism, sprains, strains, sciatica, pulled tendons and muscles, prolapsed internal organs, paralysis, and related conditions. It improves resistance to disease, increases vitality, and improves the flow of vital energy (chi).

Note: Massage must not be used on anyone suffering from fever, varicose veins, phlebitis, or thrombosis. Anyone with these conditions should seek professional health care advice.

Excessive or vigorous deep kneading massages should be avoided by people with moderate or severe lower back pain because they can injure previously damaged tissues. These types of massages are best used by experts, such as chiropractors, naturopaths, physical therapists, or masseurs. You can be injured when massaged by an inept or misguided masseur. The tissues can be aggravated and cause increased back problems. If you are unsure of your masseur's expertise, insist on a gentle stroking-type of massage until he or she builds your confidence.

There are four basic massage techniques: effleurage, petrisage, friction, and percussion. Effleurage is a stroking movement (either light or heavy); petrisage (kneading) and friction (pressure) are usually used together and are known as compression. Percussion involves a drumminglike movement.

Massage is of particular benefit for athletes or anyone doing extensive physical workouts because tendons and muscles are frequently severely strained. Also, elderly people who do not exercise vigorously particularly benefit from massage. A stroking, gentle massage is relaxing and soothing.

Sometimes, shiatsu, acupressure, trigger-point therapy, or deep pressure massage over a painful area for five to ten seconds can decrease painful local muscle spasms in both mild and moderate soft tissue conditions. If you're desperate to try, insist on a gentle, stroking type of massage. However, back off if you are not confident of your masseur.

Massaging with the use of oils helps to relieve muscle aches and back pain and helps tone muscles. Muscles often ache because of lactic acid buildup. By gradually increasing the pressure of a massage from gentle to almost the point of pain, the lactic acid can be eased out of the tissue cells and into the bloodstream. The toxins are removed, and healthy, oxygenated blood is brought to the painful tissue to speed healing. The massage should be conducted in a circular motion and always in the direction of the heart but never down toward the feet. (Also see "Aromatherapy," page 201; "Reflexology," page 216; and "Shiatsu," page 222.)

Chinese Massage Chinese massage techniques involve rubbing and pushing the ball of the thumb or the heel of the hand along the meridians, particularly those on both sides of the spine, extending from the base of the neck to the lower back and then down both legs.

The purpose of Chinese massage is to stimulate chi and the circulation of blood; clear the meridians of blockages and wastes; relax stiff muscles and loosen stiff joints; and increase resistance to disease and improve energy.

Chinese massage is frequently used in combination with acupressure, acupuncture, and moxibustion to treat muscle cramps, nervous disorders, asthma, migraine, insomnia, palpitations, shock, bursitis, fatigue, and premenstrual tension.

Massage is often used with herbal poultices and compresses on the assumption that what can't be accomplished by one treatment can be aided by others.

Note: Massage is often accompanied by the use of aromatherapy, liniments, lotions, and ointments. See discussions of these techniques in this chapter.

Massage Oils Massages are often conducted with the use of massage oils. Oils can act not only as lubricants but also as a source of health-giving essential oils. Tables 9.3 and 9.4 provide recipes for relieving muscles aches and joint pain. *Note:* Each of the herbal massage mixtures should be diluted with 50 milliliters of vegetable oil before applying.

Table 9.3

MASSAGE OILS TO RELIEVE MUSCLE ACHES

	ESSENTIAL OIL	AMOUNT
Massage oil #1	Lavender	10 drops
	Juniper	7 drops
	Rosemary	8 drops
Massage oil #2	Rosemary	11 drops
	Lavender	14 drops

Table 9.4

MASSAGE OILS TO RELIEVE JOINT PAIN

	ESSENTIAL OIL	AMOUNT
Massage oil #1	Frankincense	6 drops
	Rosemary	13 drops
	Eucalyptus	6 drops
Massage oil #2	Jasmine	5 drops
	Ylang-ylang	9 drops
	Rosewood	11 drops

Ointments

An ointment is a salve, or unction. TCM uses an ointment as a "medicine paste." Ointments are made by combining powdered herbal ingredients in a base of vegetable shortening, animal fat, or petroleum jelly. Ben-Gay, made from methyl salicylate and menthol, is one of the best-known commercial ointments for back and joint pain. Mentholatum is another topical analgesic ointment; it contains menthol and camphor in a base of petrolatum.

Ointments can be made at home quite easily. Here is an ointment recipe you might try:

Ingredients:
1 cup of shortening, petroleum jelly, or animal fat such as lard
2 tablespoons or more of herbs

To prepare:
1. Place the shortening in a 1-quart saucepan.
2. Add the herbs.
3. Bring the contents to a boil.
4. When it reaches the boiling point, turn the burner to low.
5. Allow to simmer for about ten minutes.

6. Watch the pan carefully, since overheated shortening or other fat can smoke and/or burst into flame.
7. Remove the pan from the heat and let cool.
8. Cover and let the mixture stand on the counter overnight.
9. The next day, reheat the mixture, then strain through cheesecloth or muslin to remove any foreign particles, such as bits of herbs.
10. Place the ointment in a jar or other container, cover, and store in your refrigerator or other cool storage spot. This ointment should keep for one to two months before turning rancid.

Ointment to Decrease Swelling This ointment is a natural folk remedy to decrease swelling from soft tissue back pain or arthritis in the back or joints.

Ingredients:
$1/2$ pound of dry mustard
1 pound of salt
Shortening or vegetable oil

To prepare:
1. Mix the dry mustard with the salt.
2. Add enough shortening or vegetable oil to make a heavy cream.
3. Mix thoroughly.
4. Place in a glass or ceramic jar and cover tightly.
5. Let sit overnight at room temperature before using.

To use:
1. Rub onto the swollen area until the ointment is absorbed.
2. Keep the ointment on the skin for twenty-four hours (remove earlier if irritation develops).
3. Wash off with warm water.
4. Repeat the ointment massage daily until swelling decreases.

Muscle Relaxant Rubdown This rubdown is for tight back (and any other) muscles and is supposedly a secret remedy of Eastern folk doctors.

Ingredients:
2 tablespoons of horseradish juice
1 cup of vegetable shortening or oil

To prepare:
1. Mix the above ingredients well.
2. Apply to aching muscles and joints.
3. Rub, rub, rub using gentle, but firm, finger pressure.
4. Keep on twenty-four hours, then reapply (remove earlier if irritation develops).
5. Keep the affected area warm overnight by bandaging with a woolen cloth.

Paste

A paste is a thick liquid substance made by boiling herbs in liquid until thick. In TCM, paste is used externally in the form of a poultice. (Poultices are discussed next.)

To make a paste, add 2 tablespoons of herbs (such as ginger or red pepper) to $1/2$ cup of water. Bring to a boil, then strain off the herbs and retain the liquid. Return the liquid to the heat and slowly boil until it forms a viscous and smooth paste. For flavor, add honey. This can help to disguise any bad taste. Place the paste in jars, seal, and store in a dry, cool place, such as a refrigerator or basement.

Poultice

A poultice is a dense and hot dressing that contains healing properties. Applied to the back or other areas, poultices can help decrease irritation and inflammation. In TCM, a poultice is prepared by first making a dense paste by combining hot water with powdered herbs. This paste is then spread over a piece of paper or cloth that is applied to the injured or inflamed area. Keep it tied in place for eight to ten hours. Healing vapors are formed by the heat of the body combining with the moisture of the herbs. This draws out evil chi.

Blocked meridians, arthritic joints, sprains, swellings, abscesses, and bruises are a few conditions commonly treated with herbal poultices.

Even American folk medicine uses poultices. A folk medicine poultice would be a mustard plaster or a red pepper and ginger poultice. The red pepper and ginger poultice is said to be the "miracle cure" for rheumatic and back pain.

1. Boil four to five dried and finely chopped hot red peppers in about $1/2$ cup of water. Decrease the amount of pepper if you have sensitive skin.
2. Boil the mixture until about three-quarters is left.
3. Mix the hot red pepper water with four grated nubs of ginger (each piece should be about 1 inch in length).
4. Add enough barley flour or rice to form a smooth cream.
5. Spread the cream on half of a cotton cloth.
6. Fold the second half of the cloth over the cream.
7. Place the poultice on the painful area.
8. Cover the poultice with gauze and/or plastic wrap.
9. Anchor the poultice and wrap with surgical tape.
10. Keep the poultice in place for eight to ten hours (remove immediately if the skin becomes more than a little red).

Reflexology

Reflexology, or foot massage, is based on the concept that certain areas on the bottom of your feet relate to, and can influence, different parts of the body. Massaging these areas (called zones) can help relieve and prevent health problems in the part of the body that corresponds to that zone. Reflexology is sometimes used as part of aromatherapy treatment but usually only as a diagnostic tool.

If a system, organ, gland, or tissue is impaired, the corresponding zone on the foot will be sensitive to external pressure. A tender area on the bottom of the foot can reflect an organ imbalance due to overwork, pain, stress, unhealthy lifestyle, poor emotional status, bad posture, or poor diet. This can block the flow of energy (chi) to target organs of the body. By applying systematic pressure to these zones, reflexologists can increase nerve supply and circulation of the blood in the body, thus balancing the body's energies, improving the flow of chi, and stimulating the body's own powers of healing.

Although reflexologists mainly deal with the zones of the feet, other areas of the body, including the ears and the hands, also contain reflex points.

Try the following reflexology technique for lower back pain:

- The room should be pleasant, quiet, and relaxing.
- Keep your fingernails short. Cut them if necessary.
- Wash and thoroughly dry your feet before the treatment.
- Place a sock on the foot not receiving therapy.
- Sit on a comfortable chair or stool.
- Put the foot without the sock on the thigh of your other leg (if necessary, place a pillow between the thigh and foot for support).
- Point the sole of your foot upward.
- Rub and press the area between the heel of the inner foot and the ankle bone. Regular massage and pressure to this area can decrease the duration and intensity of lower back pain. (This zone is also important for women with menstrual irregularity and pain and other problems in the pelvic area.)
- Using a massage lotion to which essential oils have been added can help increase the benefit of this technique and improve its calming and stimulating effect. For example, for relaxation, add a lavender essential oil; to help reenergize, add a rosemary essential oil.
- Massage for thirty to sixty minutes.
- Ten or more treatments may be necessary to relieve symptoms.

Trigger-Point Therapy

A trigger point is an area in a tissue that is overly irritable and tender when pressed. If very irritable, it can cause referred pain and tenderness. These trigger points affect larger areas, called target areas. By relaxing the trigger point, pain and muscle spasm are decreased or eliminated in the target area, such as the back.

Placing pressure on a trigger point helps to fatigue the muscle, causing it to relax. This technique is used with fibromyalgia, the myofascial pain syndrome, and other conditions having trigger points and target areas as described by Dr. Janet G. Travell and David G. Simons in their book *Myofascial Pain and Dysfunction*.[11] Pressure-point therapy does not involve meridians as does acupuncture, acupressure, and shiatsu, although some of the trigger points may correspond to the acupoints in TCM.

HELPFUL THERAPIES PERFORMED BY PROFESSIONALS

Certain techniques are almost impossible to perform on yourself and require another person's assistance. The following techniques are very effective at treating back pain but are best performed by trained professionals.

Acupuncture

The goal of acupuncture is to create harmony within the body by restoring the flow of chi—the life force involved in all functions of the body, including metabolism, breathing, heartbeat, and emotions.

Chi collects in organs and travels along energy channels in the body called meridians. The Chinese believe that disease occurs when the circulation of chi is stopped because of illnesses, injuries, cold, heat, and other influences. By redirecting the flow of chi, acupuncture can help cure disease, prevent illness, and restore harmony.

Acupuncture is an ancient Chinese medicine that uses small needles to penetrate the skin and stimulate the body's vital energy (qi, or chi). This energy flows between and within zones (meridians) of the body. It is believed that discomfort or disease results when this energy flow is misdirected or deranged in any way. The acupuncturist can rebalance and redirect the abnormal flow of chi by using needles to stimulate specific zonal reflex points in the body. Sterile, disposable needles should always be used to protect against the possibility of transmitting AIDS, HIV, or hepatitis.

Despite its skeptics, acupuncture is effective in treating

many conditions, both external and internal, and it is valuable in treating nervous disorders and depression. Acupuncture originated in China and is widely used throughout Asia for a variety of purposes, including pain control. Acupuncture seems to stimulate endorphin production in the body. Endorphins are morphinelike neuropeptides that can cause pain relief. When certain acupoints are stimulated, endorphins are released by the brain.

During acupuncture, the vital organs, including the brain and nervous system, are stimulated when the thin steel needles are inserted into painless nerve-ending (or vital-energy) points on the body. The stimulation of these points has specific effects on the various organs to which the points are related. In addition, acupuncture has a more universal effect on improving the body's vital energy (chi).

Adjustments or Manipulations

An adjustment is the primary technique used by chiropractors, naturopaths, and osteopaths. It is the use of mild pressure on a portion of a specific vertebra to return the vertebra to its proper position and thereby remove any nerve pressure and irritation, restore proper nerve function, and reestablish the vertebra's normal motion. This technique can reduce pain and discomfort. The doctor's training and experience, along with the nature of your problem, will determine the type of adjustment and frequency of manipulation.

Applied Kinesiology

Applied kinesiology (AK) is a popular, conservative, nonsurgical, and nondrug health care technique used by a number of chiropractors, naturopaths, medical doctors, osteopaths, dentists, and other health care providers. The technique was developed by Dr. George Goodheart. AK determines the balance or imbalance of health in the body's organs and glands by identifying specific muscle weaknesses through AK techniques. An applied kinesiologist can diagnose and resolve many health problems by relaxing or stimulating these key muscles. AK is used to maintain health and to treat degenerative back and other disorders but remains a controversial treatment program.

Goodheart apparently took traditional Eastern techniques (which activate energies in the body) and developed methods that used muscle testing and kinesiology to help identify muscle weakness, sources of dysfunction, effectiveness of treatment, and restoration of muscle balancing—essential for all health, wellness, and good posture.[12–14] He called his concept applied kinesiology.

Goodheart used applied kinesiology to diagnose and treat hypotonicity and associated hypertonic muscles. Goodheart found a reciprocal relationship between muscles—for example, between the biceps and triceps of the arm. Under normal circumstances, when one muscle contracts, the other relaxes. However, when this balance is not present, body imbalance and muscle distortion occur, resulting in such conditions as spinal curvatures, short legs, and unlevel hips. In other words, posture can indicate muscle weakness (see the discussion on posture in chapter 4).

Goodheart felt that a specific muscle weakness can reflect an organ weakness. Therefore, by testing the relative strength or weakness of a specific muscle and noting its response, one could obtain insight into the health or weakness of the related organ. Therefore, an organ or muscle weakness can be seen as back pain.

Through the use of TCM and applied kinesiology, it is hypothesized that specific muscle weaknesses can be tested and treated. The concept involves not only testing and treating muscles but much more. Goodheart conceptualized that certain muscles relate to specific organs in the body and share an acupuncture meridian. By improving muscle function, energy flow of these systems can be restored. With this approach, specific diseases, organs, or symptoms can be treated. The goal is to help the whole body help itself. It is hypothesized that by testing the muscles and by treating the muscle weaknesses, the underlying body disharmony—and not just the symptom—is being treated.

In applied kinesiology, cross-crawl is referred to as cross-patterning and is used to correct neurological disorganization. Applied kinesiologists feel that evidence of improper development may result from prolonged restrictive movement, such as arm or leg casts from a fractured bone. Further, severe health problems during neurological development may interfere with proper development. Therefore, indications are that cross-patterning helps to correct neurological function.

Cupping

Cupping (in ancient times called the "horn method") is a technique that involves creating a vacuum on selected points of the skin's surface by introducing heat, then putting a suction cup (made of glass, bamboo, or ceramic) to the skin. The theory behind this Chinese technique is that it withdraws and spreads out the evil *chi* and removes poisons.

The cupping technique is used to induce blood flow to the area and is indicated in the treatment of numerous disorders, but primarily in conditions such as arthritis (particularly in the lower back), soft tissue injuries, asthma, bronchitis, paralysis, pain in the extremities, sprains, and rheumatism and those involving bruises, swollen areas, boils, and abscesses.

Meridian Therapy

Meridian therapy is any therapy that affects the meridians through which vital energy, or chi, flows. See the sections on acupressure, acupuncture, massage, moxibustion, reflexology, and shiatsu in this chapter.

Moxibustion

Moxibustion is a form of therapy similar in effect to acupressure and acupuncture. However, in this therapy, a glowing wick (made of moxa wool) is used instead of needles to stimulate the energy points on the meridians. Igniting the moxa wool produces heat on the energy points or on specific locations of the body.

Moxa wool is made from dry mugwort or Chinese wormwood, that is, moxa leaves (*Artemesia vulgaris*) or other herbs. The herbs are ground to a fine powder and the coarse residue removed, resulting in a type of smooth "cloth." Some practitioners believe that the older the moxa wool, the better the treatment.

In the past, moxa wool was made in the shape of a cone. A small cone would be the size of a grain of wheat, while a large cone would be about $^1/_2$ inch in height and $^1/_4$ inch in diameter. Moxa wool can also be rolled into a piece about 9 inches long and $^1/_2$ inch in diameter. It can then be rolled in soft paper.

To perform moxibustion, the glowing wick is held above a vital energy point and slowly rotated. When it is performed at the same time as acupuncture, the acupuncture needles are first inserted into the skin and then the moxa piece is placed on top of the needles and ignited.

Physical Therapy (Physiotherapy)

Physical therapy (physiotherapy) is the use of natural forces such as ice, heat, light, water, massage, electricity, and exercise in the treatment of musculoskeletal diseases and joint and back pain. Chiropractors, naturopaths, osteopaths, orthopedists, physical therapists, and other health care providers all use these techniques to a greater or lesser degree to treat back pain. For an explanation of how practitioners use these modalities, see the discussion of the specific therapy.

Shiatsu

Shiatsu is a Japanese type of massage and manipulation based on ancient Asian theories concerning lines of energy (or meridians) in the body. Through shiatsu (*tsubos*, in Japanese), hundreds of acupoints can be stimulated (similar to acupressure or acupuncture). With acupressure, only the fingertips are used, while shiatsu uses thumbs, fingers, palms, knuckles, elbows, and sometimes even feet.

In 1955, the Japanese Ministry of Health and Welfare recognized shiatsu as a valid treatment.[15] Shiatsu was placed in a general category with Western-style massage and traditional Japanese massage. Illness and injuries are treated by releasing or balancing vital energy (chi), which the Japanese refer to as *ki*. Shiatsu is similar to TCM in that it is based on the concept of harmony and balance—that all energies are either yin (cold, negative, inactive) or yang (hot, positive, active), which complement each other. Illness is either internal (*kyo*) or external (*jitsu*).

Ultrasound

Generally speaking, ultrasound causes a deep heating of the tissue, relaxes muscle spasms, increases the flow of blood, relieves pain, and removes waste products. An ultrasound unit produces mechanical radiant energy and vibrates at a frequency above that which can be heard by the human ear (greater than 20,000 cycles per second). This helps the energy to penetrate into the deeper layers of tissue. Ultrasound is the preferred treatment in most painful disorders, especially those resulting from damaged ligaments and soft tissues.

Ultrasound is very effective in the treatment of rheumatoid arthritis and osteoarthritis, bursitis, fibrositis, neuritis, sprains and strains, tendonitis, and tender trigger points. It is contraindicated in a number of conditions (such as acute infections and vascular diseases) and over certain areas of the body (such as over the eyes, heart, reproductive organs, or brain).

Ten

Treating Specific Conditions That Cause Back Pain

The techniques listed in chapters 7, 8, and 9 of this book are effective in treating the majority of painful back conditions, such as sprains and strains, muscle soreness, and nerve problems. However, back pain can also occur because of a specific health condition, such as arthritis, fibromyalgia, osteoporosis, or other illness. This chapter outlines specific treatment plans and gives you the ammunition to fight specific conditions that cause back pain.

Each and every back condition requires use of the Five-Step Jump-Start Plus Program—that is, meditation and a positive mental attitude, physical exercise (the level depends on the condition and seriousness of the condition), and of course nutrition. Fasting, juicing, diet, and supplements are all essential. Everyone should take multivitamin, multimineral, and multienzyme supplements for general health. In addition to the specific supplements listed in this chapter for each condition, take the supplements and herbs discussed in chapter 8 to improve bone strength, muscle strength, flexibility, circulation, and immune function and to control inflammation.

This chapter explains the additional emotional, nutritional, and physical steps you can take if you suffer from a health condition whose symptoms include back pain. Only information for each specific condition will be noted in this chapter. See chapters 7, 8, and 9 for general guidelines relating to the treatment of back pain.

It is important to be flexible when treating the conditions that can cause back pain. These conditions and their symptoms may change and vary from week to week or even from day to day. You are special! You are a unique person with special needs and problems. Therefore, it is wise to be flexible in treating back pain and be prepared to continually evaluate and reevaluate the symptoms and treatment programs.

The conditions discussed in this chapter involve a wide variety of symptoms, such as acute or chronic pain, inflammation, swelling, muscle stiffness and soreness, numbness, limited movement, and joint deformity. However, pain and restricted movement are the symptoms most common to back problems.

If you suffer from one of the conditions described in this chapter, it is wise to seek the services of a well-trained conservative back specialist.

ANKYLOSING SPONDYLITIS

When Bridget was twenty-five years old, she was full of vim, vigor, and vitality. Although her lower back was sometimes a little stiff, activity usually made the pain go away. Her physician took X rays, but everything appeared normal. Unfortunately, as she aged, the pain and stiffness worsened. I first saw Bridget when at age fifty-five she came to my office complaining of constant back pain. Back X rays and a bone scan confirmed the diagnosis of ankylosing spondylitis (AS).

Ankylosing spondylitis is a rheumatic disorder that is believed to be genetic, although environmental factors or immune system malfunction may also influence its development. It usually begins when a person is between twenty and forty years of age, and it affects men three times more often than women.[1]

My orthopedic colleagues and I have seen many cases of

this condition with its devastating effects. Two elderly women in their late eighties come to mind. Their spines were severely curved forward, and the vertebrae had fused in that position. The curvature was so great that they were unable to raise their heads and were forced to look at the ground as they spoke.

This "hunched-over" posture can lead to other problems, because as the individual is forced to bend forward, there is a decrease in both lung capacity and in the size of the cavity that houses various vital organs. Another complicating problem can be spontaneous fractures of the spinal vertebrae, thus weakening the spine and further decreasing abdominal cavity size. Subluxations, sciatica, and a condition called *cauda equina syndrome* can also develop. The cauda equina is the lowest portion of the spinal cord. The group of nerves that leaves the spine through openings in the sacrum resembles a horse's tail—thus the name cauda equina, which literally means "horse's tail." Cauda equina syndrome is a neurological condition that can result in urinary incontinence (particularly at night), impotency, decreased sensation in the rectal and bladder area, and a decrease in the nerve and blood supply to the cauda equina area.

Anyone suffering from ankylosing spondylitis should be under the care of a well-trained physician. In addition to massage, physical therapy, nutritional guidance, and (possibly) chiropractic adjustments, your physician may also show you techniques for proper lifting, bending, walking, and other body movements to help you avoid injury. To help this condition, follow the suggestions in the section on arthritis.

ARTHRITIS

In the Western world, the two major types of arthritis are osteoarthritis and rheumatoid arthritis. Osteoarthritis is an inflammatory problem that primarily affects the weight-bearing joints, such as the spine, hips, sacroiliac, and knees. In this disease, the protective joint cartilage at the ends of bones gradually wears away. This occurs particularly in the spine and legs. Without the protective cartilage, the surface of the bones becomes exposed, and the bones rub together.

This can cause bone spurs to develop, which can damage nerves and muscles and lead to bone deformity, pain, and restricted movement.

Rheumatoid arthritis (RA) is a chronic inflammatory condition that specifically affects the synovial membranes of the joints but can also involve the entire body. RA is an autoimmune disease—that is, the body's immune system is attacking the body itself. It is a condition associated with elevated levels of immune complexes circulating in the blood.

Although its onset may be abrupt, RA usually begins gradually. It can begin at any age, but the average age of onset is between twenty and forty. Approximately 1 percent of Americans are affected by RA, and females outnumber males by a margin of nearly three to one.[2] The joints typically involved in this disease are the spine, feet, hands, knees, ankles, and wrists. Characteristic symptoms include vague joint pain, joint stiffness, low-grade fever, fatigue, and general weakness that can appear several weeks before the onset of swollen and painful joints.

Rheumatoid arthritis and osteoarthritis are frequently frustrating to treat. One of the problems is that symptoms can vary from one week—or even one day—to the next. Also, environmental temperature and humidity can cause varied symptoms. For instance, mornings can be wet and cold producing one set of symptoms, while the afternoon may become dry and hot, producing yet another set of symptoms.

As is the case with many health conditions, the Chinese see arthritis in a totally different light. In Traditional Chinese Medicine (TCM), arthritis is called *bi*, or "blockage" syndrome. The blockage syndrome relates to the presence of four evils (cold, wind, damp, and heat) that invade the body and joints, blocking the flow of chi and blood. The result is painful joints.

The four evils correspond to the four groups of arthritis: damp, wind, heat, and cold types. Each has its own symptomatology.

- *Damp type*. This type is characterized by lingering and aching dull pain, swelling, stiffness, sluggishness, and a feeling of heaviness. Overweight and obese individuals with arthritis usually have this type.

- *Wind type.* This type of arthritis is characterized by shifting pain that can suddenly come and go (similar to the wind). Sufferers may also have occasional dizziness.
- *Heat type.* This type is characterized by painful, swollen, hot, red joints, usually of acute onset and generally disabling.
- *Cold type.* This type is characterized by coldness of the joints with stabbing and sharp pain in specific locations.

The Five-Step Jump-Start Plus Program can effectively treat arthritis, regardless of its cause or type. Because arthritis affects the whole body, it is important to treat it holistically by integrating emotional, nutritional, and physical techniques. In addition to the therapies outlined in chapters 7, 8, and 9, adhere to the following guidelines.

Emotional Techniques

- Help your body to reenergize by meditating at least fifteen minutes every day. Meditation can help you keep a positive mental attitude—especially important when your arthritis pain starts to get you down.
- Be sure to get adequate rest.
- Be sensitive to your own symptoms and how they react to changes in climate.

Nutritional Techniques

- Take chondroitin sulfate (250 milligrams, two or three times per day) or glucosamine sulfate/hydrochloride (500 milligrams, two to four times per day). These beneficial nutrients stimulate cartilage repair and nourish connective tissue.
- Take adequate calcium (1,000 milligrams per day) and magnesium (500 milligrams per day). These minerals play important roles in the proper contraction of muscles and in the function of nerves.
- Sufficient vitamin C (1,000 to 10,000 milligrams per day) can help the delivery of oxygen to the cells and aid

in the production of collagen and normal connective tissue. This vitamin bolsters the immune system and is a potent antioxidant.

- Cut down on your intake of calories and fat. You may find that eliminating dairy products and meat helps reduce your symptoms.
- There is some indication that members of the nightshade family, such as eggplant, peppers, potatoes, and tomatoes, may aggravate arthritis symptoms.
- To treat rheumatoid arthritis, increase your intake of alpha-linolenic acid (found in walnuts, flaxseed, and soy products). This important nutrient can reduce inflammation. Also eat more salmon, tuna, and other cold-water fish, rich in eicosapentaenoic acid (EPA), effective in the treatment of rheumatoid arthritis.
- A number of herbs can be beneficial. Drink decoctions and infusions of angelica root, mulberry leaves, fang feng root, cinnamon bark, and Job's tears.
- Proteolytic enzymes are effective in fighting all forms of arthritis because they can fight inflammation and relieve pain. In one study on RA, forty-two patients with RA were treated with a mixture of enzymes (containing pancreatin, papain, bromelain, lipase, amylase, trypsin, chymotrypsin, and rutin) for a minimum of six weeks.[3] After enzyme treatment, twenty-six (61.9 percent) of the patients had improved, thirteen (30.9 percent) were unchanged, and the condition of three (7.1 percent) had deteriorated. No side effects were observed.
- A beneficial herbal tea remedy could include 6 grams each of achyranthes (niu xi), angelica (dang qui), cinnamon bark (rou giu), asarum (xi xin), eucommia (du zhong), ginseng (ren shen), gentian (qin jaio), ligusticum (chuan xiong), mistletoe (san ji sheng), sileris (fang feng), rehmannia (shen di huang), and honey-fried licorice (zhi gan cao) along with 8 grams of poria (fu ling) and 9 grams of angelica root (duo duo). This tea should be divided into at least three servings and taken between meals.
- For damp-type arthritis, suggested foods include barley,

cornsilk tea, millet, mung beans, mustard greens, red beans, and sweet rice wine with meat. Especially therapeutic is a mixture of mung beans, red beans, and barley. Avoid dairy products and cold foods.

- For wind-type arthritis, suggested foods include black beans, grape vine, grapes (not wine), green leafy vegetables, most grains, mulberry vine tea, and scallions. Avoid alcohol, meat, shellfish, smoking, stimulants, and sugar.
- For heat-type arthritis, suggested foods include cabbage, dandelion, fresh fruits and vegetables (as much as possible), mung beans, soybean sprouts, and winter melon. Avoid alcohol, green onions, smoking, spicy foods, and stress.
- For cold-type arthritis, suggested foods include black beans, chicken, garlic, ginger, grape vine, grapes, green onion, lamb, mustard greens, parsnips, pepper, sesame seeds, and spicy foods.

Physical Techniques

- Exercise can help increase circulation and keep the joints more flexible. Water exercises are particularly beneficial because they remove the pull of gravity and take pressure off the joints. Warm water can also help the muscles to relax. If you suffer from osteoarthritis, at first the pain may increase with exercise. But stick with it. Exercise can actually improve the stiffness that may occur because of inactivity. Follow the exercises in chapter 9, beginning with the level 1 exercises and increasing the level of difficulty as your back and body tell you. If you are seeing a back specialist, ask for his or her advice.
- Warm (or hot) packs can help relax muscles and relieve joint stiffness and pain.
- Topical applications of DMSO (dimethylsulfoxide) diluted in equal parts of water may be helpful in reducing your pain, improving circulation, and removing toxins.
- Acupuncture, acupressure, and moxibustion can stimulate meridians (particularly the kidney, gallbladder, large intestine, and stomach meridians), nourish the joints, and improve circulation.

- Massage can help relieve the painful symptoms of arthritis. A lotion of sesame oil mixed with powdered rhizome of rhubarb (*Rheum officinale*) can be used with massage.
- An effective liniment can be made by combining 1 tablespoon of cayenne pepper with 1 pint of apple cider vinegar or rice vinegar. Place in a saucepan on medium heat. Cover and simmer for ten minutes (do not boil). Pour into a bottle and seal while still hot. When cool, rub the liniment gently into the skin.
- Cold-type arthritis may respond to the external application of scallion tea, ginger, garlic, or rice wine.

DISK PROBLEMS (ACUTE DISK SYNDROME, "SLIPPED DISK")

George was playing soccer when he kicked the ball and immediately felt a sharp, stabbing pain across his lower back, particularly on the left side, with a sharp shooting pain down the back of his left leg to his heel. His lower back hurt when he coughed or sneezed. He could not walk on the balls of his feet, and his heels dropped to the floor with every step. Bent to the right and slightly forward, George could only move his feet in short shuffling steps. As he entered the office, he dropped to his knees and crawled several feet before finally collapsing to the floor. It was impossible for him to stand in an upright position. George had a protruded (slipped) disk.

The disk is a fibrous cushion that acts to pad and maintain the space between the twenty-four movable vertebrae. These twenty-three cushionlike pillows make flexibility of the spine possible (and are critical for normal movement) but act in much the same way as shock absorbers in a car or the springs in your mattress. Your disks are constantly under stress—expanding and compressing, turning, twisting, and torquing.

Injury can cause pressure and trauma to the outer portion of the disk, allowing the inner portion (the nucleus pulposis—the "jelly" in the doughnut) to ooze out and place pressure on nearby nerves and arteries. This pressure can cause debilitating pain.

Warning: If a disk problem is suspected, see a physician immediately for examination, consultation, and treatment. The longer you wait, the more serious could be the consequences. However, surgery is not always necessary. Often, this condition can be successfully treated with conservative methods, such as those of the Five-Step Jump-Start Plus Program.

You can begin the emotional and nutritional therapies in this book immediately. The back exercises in this book will help promote flexibility and strengthen your back and also improve circulation. However, exercises can aggravate a severe disk problem, so no back exercise should be initiated without a doctor's approval.

Emotional Techniques

■ Choose any meditation technique in chapter 7. Visualization is a good technique to meditate on the disk repairing itself, the waste products leaving the injured area, and healthy blood and chi coming to the area to speed healing.

Nutritional Techniques

■ Good nutrition is essential to decrease any inflammation, remove the waste products, improve circulation, and strengthen the disk and surrounding tissue.

■ It is essential that you take high doses of proteolytic enzymes (such as bromelain and serratiopeptidase) to reduce inflammation and swelling, improve circulation, and speed healing. Be sure to take them between meals.

■ Vitamin C is important to help produce collagen and normal connective tissue. It is also a potent antioxidant. Take at least 8,000 milligrams per day until your pain resolves.

■ To increase oxygen delivery to the cells and therefore speed recovery, take adequate vitamin E (at least 1,200 IU per day).

■ Take ginger capsules (250 milligrams three times per day). Ginger contains zingibain, a powerful proteolytic enzyme.

■ The herb kava kava can promote sleep and induce

relaxation. Kava kava may also have an analgesic effect. Take 250 milligrams three times per day.

- Turmeric contains curcumin, which is effective at fighting inflammation and pain. Take 250 milligrams three times per day.
- Boswellia can reduce inflammation and improve blood supply to the joints. Take 250 milligrams three times per day.
- Take 15 to 20 milligrams of yucca three times per day to fight inflammation and enhance healing.
- Devil's claw fights inflammation, relieves pain, and relaxes muscles. Take 15 to 20 milligrams three times per day.
- The flavonoid quercetin fights inflammation, reduces capillary fragility, and stabilizes membranes. Take 15 to 20 milligrams three times per day.

Physical Techniques

- Avoid exercising until your physician gives you the "go ahead." Then, with your doctor's approval, begin with the level 1 exercises in chapter 9.
- Icing the affected area can help reduce swelling and pain.

FIBROMYALGIA (MYOFASCIAL PAIN SYNDROME, FIBROMYOSITIS)

Stan worked at a computer all day and was constantly under tremendous pressure. As each day progressed, Stan could feel the tension in his neck, shoulders, and upper back mounting. The pain was exquisite and sometimes unbearable. Ethel, Stan's wife, tried to massage his back, but he screamed in pain. There were specific "trigger points" that, when pressed, caused pain in other areas of his back (these are called "target areas"). Stan suffers from fibromyalgia.

Fibromyalgia refers to a group of chronic, rheumatic, soft tissue conditions whose symptoms include achy tenderness, pain, and muscle stiffness where the muscle tendons insert into bones and in adjacent soft tissue areas. Any of the fibromuscular tissues can be affected, but those of the occiput (the bone at the base of the skull), neck, shoulders, thorax, lower back, and thighs are most common. Fibromyalgia may cause chronic lower back stiffness and pain and may be associated with well-defined tender points, fatigue, muscle strain, stress, anxiety, or nonrestorative sleep, with or without inflammation. Fibromyalgia can be caused or worsened by stress of any kind, poor sleep, injury, viruses and other infections, and exposure to cold or damp conditions.

In TCM, soft tissue back pain is associated with blood deficiency, an imbalance in the liver and spleen, a deficiency of chi, or stagnation in liver chi. Excessive stress, areas of extreme pain, constipation or loose bowels, insomnia, fatigue, and hot arms and legs can be indications of liver or spleen imbalance. A dull, aching pain or sharp, stabbing pain indicates involvement of blood and chi.

Emotional Techniques

- Emotional stress is a common factor in fibromyalgia. To help relieve stress, practice the relaxation exercises in chapter 7.
- Use visualization techniques to visualize the pain diminishing and leaving the affected areas. Visualize the painful area as feeling heavy. This will help to reduce muscle tension.

Nutritional Techniques

- Take calcium (at least 1,000 milligrams per day) and magnesium (at least 500 milligrams per day) to aid muscle contraction and nerve transmission.
- Take 250 milligrams of chondroitin sulfate (two or three times per day with meals) to support connective tissue; nourish cartilage, ligaments, and tendons; and promote cell hydration.
- Fibromyalgia sufferers typically have difficulty sleeping. Herbs, including valerian, can help you to relax and get a good night's rest. Take 190 milligrams a half hour before retiring.
- Ginger tea can help relieve pain and improve circulation. Boil a piece of gingerroot (or several slices) in a cup of water for about ten minutes. Drink two or three times per day.

- You might try the following TCM remedies to combat fibromyalgia:
    - Combine sesame seeds (30 grams) with walnut seeds (30 grams). Grind the seeds to a powder. Mix with $^1/_2$ to 1 cup of water. Drink the liquid once daily.
    - Date remedy relieves blood and chi deficiency pain. In a saucepan, combine 60 pieces of Chinese dates with 2 raw, whole eggs and 50 grams of dry logan (long yan rou). Cook over medium heat until the dates are soft. Drink half of the above mixture two times a day between meals.
    - Rice or barley congee (porridge) with herbs decreases blood stasis and improves circulation. To prepare, combine 1 cup of rice with 5 or 6 cups of water in a heavy-lidded ceramic pot. Simmer over the lowest flame or electrical current possible for four to six hours. Add a decoction or tea that consists of peach seeds (with tip and skin removed) (10 grams), rehmannia root (2 grams), and unrefined brown sugar (50 grams). Drink 1 cup twice per day between meals.

Physical Techniques

- The stretching exercises in chapter 9 can help you to stretch and relax your muscles.
- A hot shower with a pulsating shower head, a hot tub, or other hydrotherapy can help relax back muscles and other areas of soft tissue tension.
- Massaging the tender areas can help, but massage may be difficult to perform on yourself.
- To effectively treat fibromyalgia, you must interrupt the pain cycle. Reflexology and trigger-point therapy can help to achieve this goal. See chapter 9 for a description of these techniques.
- Apply a comfrey and vinegar poultice. This poultice can be helpful for muscle back pain. Vinegar improves blood flow, and comfrey helps the injured area heal. To make, mash a handful of dried or fresh comfrey leaves and soak

with enough nondistilled vinegar (such as apple cider vinegar) to thoroughly soak the comfrey. Make a paste. Place the mash directly on the painful area (at least $^{1}/_{2}$ inch thick). Cover with a clean cotton cloth (secure, but not too tight). *Note:* If comfrey is not available, use spinach, plantain, cabbage, or chard leaves.

- Another effective poultice can be made by combining 9 grams each of tang kuei and red peony with 6 grams each of peach kernel, safflower, ginseng, frankincense, and myrrh and 1 cup of water in a small saucepan. Simmer over medium heat for two to three minutes. Soak a thin, warm washcloth in the herbal liquid and place it on the painful area, or put the wet herbs on a thin warm cloth (muslin or other loosely woven cloth) and fold over the herbs and place the cloth on the inflamed and painful area for up to twenty-four hours, or as needed. Keep the poultice warm and comfortable. When it begins to cool, change the poultice.

- A chive poultice can help decrease pain and swelling and can decrease blood coagulation and increase blood flow. Finely chop the roots and leaves of chives and wring them through muslin or juice them in a juicer. Soak a cotton cloth in the resulting liquid. Place the cloth on the injured area and keep warm and comfortable.

- Other poultices to help decrease back pain include those made from charcoal and lobelia, goldenseal, or mustard.

- Your physician has a number of therapies at his or her disposal to help interrupt the pain cycle. These include manipulation, massage, pressure-point therapy, ultrasound, electrical stimulation, and a technique called "stretch and spray." In this technique, a coolant such as ethyl chloride is sprayed over the painful area and the skin is then stretched.

- Acupressure and acupuncture can be effective in treating fibromyalgia. The points chosen relate to the symptoms and would be primarily used to treat a chi deficiency, a blood deficiency, a liver and spleen imbalance, or liver chi stagnation.

OSTEOARTHRITIS (SEE ARTHRITIS, PAGE 227)

OSTEOPOROSIS

As Margaret aged, her children moved out, her husband died, and she lived alone. She stopped eating a well-balanced diet, quit taking her supplements, and no longer exercised. One morning, as Margaret got out of bed, her right hip gave way and she collapsed painfully to the floor. She was rushed to the hospital, examined, and diagnosed as having a fracture of the right hip, caused by osteoporosis.

Osteoporosis (meaning "porous bones") is a condition marked by deterioration of the spinal vertebrae or the weight-bearing joints, such as the hips. It is usually diagnosed only after a person fractures a hip or one or more of the vertebrae collapse (this is called a compression fracture). This condition affects women much more frequently (two to six times) than men.[4]

In this condition, bones gradually thin and weaken, a process that leaves them highly susceptible to fractures. It is marked by a loss of bone mass. Found predominantly in those forty-five years of age and older, this condition affects some fifteen to twenty million Americans, causing an estimated 1.3 million fractures (every year) of the vertebrae, forearms, hips, and other bones.[4]

Of particular importance are dietary factors relating to osteoporosis. These nutrients are vitamin D, phosphate, and calcium. Calcium will be pulled from the bones and teeth if calcium levels are not sufficient. This contributes to osteoporosis as well as dental problems. To help prevent osteoporosis, many physicians prescribe hormone replacement therapy (HRT). This is probably because calcium absorption increases with estrogen intake.

But hormone replacement therapy may also increase your chance of suffering from back pain. A recent study by Brynhildsen and colleagues found that women who received HRT experienced a significant increase in back pain compared with those not receiving HRT.[5] These findings could not be explained by differences in current physical activity, smoking habits, or occupation. The researchers speculated that the difference in findings might involve the hormonal effects on ligaments and joints.

As we age, our diet and exercise are often neglected, and our body continues to deteriorate. However, if caught in its early stages, osteoporosis can be effectively treated. The Five-Step Jump-Start Plus Program is an excellent way to combine TCM with Western treatment to combat osteoporosis. Regular exercise, meditation, a positive mental attitude, and proper nutrition are all essential.

Emotional Techniques

- A regular daily program of meditation helps reduce stress and improve body harmony, balance, and the flow of chi.

Nutritional Techniques

- Eat plenty of calcium-rich foods, including yogurt, cheese, milk, and other dairy products. Other sources of calcium include oily fish and some vegetables (such as spinach, sweet potatoes, and tomatoes).
- Be sure to eat enough vitamin D foods, such as fatty fish, eggs, and margarine.
- Decrease your intake of alcohol, salt, and meat.
- In TCM, osteoporosis is described as a condition of kidney deficiency and may be treated as such.
- Drink a decoction or infusion of 8 to 15 grams of Eucommia bark (*Eucommia ulmoides*) twice daily between meals. Eucommia acts as a sedative and analgesic and is said to fortify the bones, tendons, and cartilage.
- Take mucopolysaccharides, such as those found in shark cartilage. These nutrients help enhance the body's normal inflammatory response, keep joint membranes fluid, and support healthy, flexible joints.

Physical Techniques

- Exercises can help you retain bone mass. Begin with the stretching and flexibility exercises (level 1) in chapter 9, and work up slowly and gradually to include qi gong, yoga, and tai chi (if possible).

- Acupuncture and acupressure on the kidney meridian are effective.

RHEUMATOID ARTHRITIS (SEE ARTHRITIS, PAGE 227)

SCIATICA

Mary fell off a horse, landing on her hips and lower back. The following morning, she felt a sharp, stabbing pain in her lower back accompanied by a sharp, shooting pain that traveled down the back of her left leg. Mary is suffering from sciatica, so named because the pain follows the sciatic nerve. The sciatic nerve is the longest nerve in the peripheral nervous system. It extends through the buttocks and down each leg as far as the ankle and foot. Sometimes, pain can occur along the entire length of the sciatic nerve.

Sciatica is not a condition by itself but rather a symptom of one or many underlying conditions. Usually, sciatica is caused by pressure on the sciatic nerve in the lumbosacral region. Frequent causes of sciatica include an acute or degenerative disk condition, spondylolisthesis, rheumatoid arthritis or osteoarthritis, muscle strain, poor posture, overweight, and pregnancy. This symptom can also result from sleeping on a mattress that is too soft or from wearing high heels.

If you suffer from sciatica, it is especially important that you see a physician. It is most likely that your symptoms are caused by a back problem; however, in rare instances, sciatica can result from extraspinal causes, such as a circulatory problem (internal iliac artery aneurysm).[6]

Emotional Techniques
- The relaxation techniques in chapter 7 can help relax the muscle spasms that can occur because of sciatica.

Nutritional Techniques
- Take an infusion of feverfew leaves, 2 to 3 grams taken internally.

- Herbs such as echinacea, gingerroot, ginkgo biloba, licorice, and white willow bark can fight inflammation and help relieve pain.
- The herb valerian is often used as a sleep aid because of its sedative action. It is effective in treating nervous tension, anxiety, and muscle pain.
- If you are overweight, you should begin a weight loss program. This will help decrease the pressure on the vertebrae.
- Be sure to take sufficient calcium (at least 1,000 milligrams every day) and magnesium (500 milligrams every day). These minerals play important roles in muscle contraction and nerve function and transmission.

Physical Techniques
- Place a hot compress or a hot-water bottle on the affected leg and a cold compress on the lower back. Leave the compresses in place for five minutes, then remove for five minutes, then reapply. Repeat this process three times in a row, three times a day.
- Apply a poultice or compress made from crushed capsules of corn poppy (*Papaver rhocas*) or crushed black mustard seeds (*Brassica nigra*). Leave in place a minimum of two hours. This will relieve pain and relax muscles.
- Acupressure and acupuncture can be used to unblock the meridians (heat and wind). The acupoints to be stimulated are those on the meridians associated with the liver, gallbladder, kidneys, stomach, and large intestine.

SCOLIOSIS

One day, Patricia, a young teenage girl, was looking in a full-length mirror and noticed that her dress hem was higher on the right side than on the left. She often experienced pain and stiffness in her neck and shoulders as well as her midback and lower back. But it was only when her mother noticed that Patricia's right shoulder and hip were higher than the left that they knew something was wrong and rushed to my office.

X rays confirmed that Patricia had an S-type curvature of the spine, or scoliosis, a condition commonly observed in children and teenagers (girls more than boys). The spine can also curve to one side, forming a C shape. Interestingly, it is not the back pain itself but more often comments from family, friends, or the mirror that drive a person to action.

Scoliosis can be caused by emotional, nutritional, physical, or unknown stressors, but it is probably the most obvious sign of disharmony and body imbalance. Emotional stress can result in muscle tension, pulling the vertebrae in one direction or the other. Nutritional disharmony can be caused by impaired digestion, absorption, or metabolism of various essential nutrients (such as calcium, magnesium, enzymes, and amino acids). Physical disharmonies include one short leg, back muscles that are in spastic imbalance, and wedged vertebrae.

Scoliosis can be either structural (involving the vertebrae) or nonstructural, in which case it can often be corrected by improving the individual's posture. Structural scoliosis can be congenital but is generally not considered genetic.

Regardless of the cause, scoliosis can put added stress on the body and cause back pain. Nerves that pass through openings between the vertebrae and transmit messages to the body and to the brain may be irritated or even pinched. Disks, the shock absorbers of the spine located between the vertebrae, may wear down, rupture, or bulge. The muscles may become weak on one side of the body and overused or tight on the other side; the base of the spine (called the sacrum) may be tilted and not level. If scoliosis persists into adult life, it can worsen and may affect adjacent organs in the body, such as the lungs and heart.

The key to effective scoliosis care is early detection. This is the purpose of preschool and grade school screenings, since scoliosis can begin to develop in early childhood years. The earlier a scoliosis is diagnosed and treated, the better the chances of controlling the curvature and stopping its progress.

Screening for Scoliosis

To be examined for scoliosis, stand straight but relaxed, with your head up. Look straight ahead, with your back to the examiner. Your feet should be together, your arms hanging down at your sides. Scoliosis may be indicated if:

- The ears or bones at the base of the skull (the occiput) are not level.
- One shoulder or hip is higher than the other.
- One scapula (shoulder blade) is more prominent than the other.
- One hand seems closer to the floor than the other.
- The legs are different lengths. To check, place the palms of your hands on each hipbone and look into a mirror. If one hand is higher than the other, you may have scoliosis.
- While bending over from the waist, one side of the back is higher than the other.

Anyone with scoliosis should be under the care of a well-trained back specialist. The earlier scoliosis is discovered, the earlier treatment can be initiated. Early treatment can help prevent the condition from worsening. The following techniques can augment your physician's therapy program.

Emotional Techniques
- Daily meditation and relaxation exercises are essential to help relax spasming muscles (see chapter 7).

Nutritional Techniques
- Nutritionally, it's back to basics. Read and reread chapter 8. Take a broad-spectrum vitamin, mineral, and enzyme supplement.
- Be sure and take glucosamine sulfate, chondroitin sulfate, and possibly methylsulfonylmethane (MSM), amino acids, L-glutamine, magnesium, calcium, and malic acid.
- Herbs such as valerian, kava kava, and passionflower can help you relax and get the rest you need.
- Proteolytic enzymes (including bromelain, papain, pancreatin, and possibly microbial proteases) can help fight inflammation and the resulting pain. A very effective enzyme combination includes bromelain, papain, pancreatin, trypsin, and chymotrypsin with the bioflavonoid rutin (see chapter 8).

- Mucopolysaccharides, such as those found in shark cartilage, can enhance the body's normal inflammatory response and support strong, flexible joints.
- If you are overweight, begin a weight loss program to decrease pressure on the spine.

Physical Techniques

- A daily program of stretching exercises is essential—emphasize joint flexibility. My back stretches in chapter 9 are good. Begin with level 1 exercises, including stretching, yoga, and qi gong exercises.
- Pressure-point therapy is beneficial to relax the muscles on the concave side of the spine and tighten the muscles on the convex side.
- Other beneficial physical techniques may include back massage or shiatsu, acupuncture, acupressure, moxibustion, and electrical stimulation. Shoe lifts can also help improve a scoliosis.
- Back supports can be helpful in many cases to prevent the scoliosis from progressing, to decrease any adverse forces, to apply corrective mechanical forces, and to stimulate corrective neuromuscular force. However, if the curve is greater than 40 degrees, back supports have little effect.
- Contact a conservative back care physician for examination and consultation. Adjustments and therapy can be very helpful. Your physician can train you in proper techniques to follow in lifting, bending, standing, sitting, sleeping, walking, and driving.

SHORT-LEG SYNDROME

Mark had a short right leg. His hips tilted low on the right, and he wore out the soles and heels of his right shoe faster than those of the left shoe. His right pant leg had to be shortened or it would drape over his right shoe. Because his hip was low on the right, he developed a compensatory curve in his spine with resulting back pain.

Short-leg syndrome is the condition in which one leg

(from the femur to the bottom of the heel) is shorter than the other. Usually first noticeable in children during their growth period, this condition can result from the overgrowth of one leg versus the other. Short-leg syndrome can also result from muscle imbalance.

Uneven skirt length or pant length or a slanted belt line are major clues of a short leg, as are shoe heels or soles that wear unevenly. Even if you don't suspect that your child has a short leg, get a screening in the early years of life.

Short-Leg Syndrome Self-Test

To see if you have a short leg, perform the following self-test:

1. Face a full-length mirror. Place your hands on your hips. Your hands should be level. If one is higher than the other, it may indicate a short leg.
2. Lie on your back on the floor with the soles of your feet flat on the floor and your knees bent at a 90-degree angle. Place a yardstick on the top of both knees. If the yardstick is slanted, it may indicate that one knee is lower than the other and thus one leg is shorter than the other.

If you suspect that you have a short leg, see a physician for evaluation and treatment. Don't try to deal with this by yourself.

SUBLUXATIONS

Got a "kink" in your neck or a "catch" in your lower back? What causes your neck to be so stiff? Why does your back hurt so much? A spinal subluxation could be the culprit.

A subluxation is an incomplete or partial dislocation of one or more vertebrae. It occurs when a vertebra is out of alignment beyond its normal range of motion and cannot return on its own. A subluxation can cause a decrease in the opening (foramen) through which the nerve passes from the spine to the body. This places pressure on the nerve and results in a decrease in nerve supply as well as pain and possible loss of function.

Subluxations can occur from injuries or other sudden

trauma or from standing or sitting for extended periods of time, poor posture, congenital problems (spinal problems existing since birth), and even pregnancy or delivery. Also, they can be the underlying cause of a scoliosis.

My Five-Step Jump-Start Plus Program is essential in treating subluxations to strengthen and balance the bones and surrounding soft tissue (muscles and ligaments) and bring harmony to the body as a whole.

Chiropractic doctors are trained to deal with subluxations. Adjustments and manipulations can help return your vertebrae to their proper positions and relieve back pain.

Emotional Techniques

■ Meditation can improve your mental attitude and help you to better cope with pain.

■ The positive mental attitude techniques in chapter 7 can help you to relax, thereby relaxing the muscles that are contracting and causing you pain.

■ Visualization techniques can help you visualize the vertebra(e) moving into alignment.

■ Subluxations often involve inflammation, which causes heat. Visualizing the area as being "cool" can help relieve discomfort.

Nutritional Techniques

■ Chondroitin sulfate and glucosamine sulfate/hydrochloride can stimulate cartilage repair, support connective tissue, promote cell hydration, and nourish the cartilage, ligaments, and tendons.

■ Take supplemental vitamin B. The B vitamins support neuromusculoskeletal function.

■ Eat plenty of vitamin C–rich foods or take supplements (1,000 to 10,000 milligrams per day). Vitamin C, in addition to being a potent antioxidant, is necessary for normal connective tissue and collagen production.

■ Herbs to fight inflammation include echinacea, gingerroot, ginkgo biloba, licorice, and white willow bark.

Physical Techniques

■ Exercises, including walking, bicycling, and swimming, can help stimulate circulation and speed your recovery. However, your ability to exercise will depend on the severity and location of your subluxation. If in doubt, consult with your physician.

Eleven

Back Pain Prevention

One summer back in the 1960s, I was teaching child behavior in the Department of Educational Psychology at the University of Georgia in Athens, Georgia. Because we were only going to be there for the summer, my wife and I decided to lease a very nice house in Athens. We had only been in Athens for a few days when the front doorbell rang. It was the local exterminator, who explained that he was there to do routine maintenance. My wife said, "But we don't have any bugs." After all, it was a mansion! He responded, "And the reason you don't have bugs is because I keep it that way." We gratefully allowed him to enter and do his job.

Back pain is a lot like the bugs that would have attacked our house that summer had we not taken steps to prevent them. We can beat them back this year, but they'll come back next year with a vengeance. *Prevention* is the key word with bugs, just as *prevention* is the key word with back pain.

Many individuals who recover from their first episode of an acute back problem will have a second episode within a few years. Unless you have new symptoms or a new medical condition that differs from the initial episode, you can expect to recover quickly and completely. Remember, however, that as you age, your body will not respond as quickly. For this reason, you should emphasize an overall healthy lifestyle and follow the prevention techniques given in this chapter.

HOW CAN YOU PREVENT BACK PAIN?

- Balance and harmony are the keys to a healthier, happier, pain-free life.
- Have a positive mental attitude. Take time to relax and smell the roses (as discussed in chapter 7).
- Make meditation and visualization a part of your daily life.
- Eat a nutritious diet and take supplements, including vitamins, minerals, enzymes, and herbs (see chapter 8).
- Keep your muscles flexible and strong (see chapter 9). Use safe stretching and strengthening exercises daily.
- Like a river of life, maintain and balance the flow of energy (chi) in your body by performing a daily program of yoga, qi gong, tai chi, tae-bo, or aerobic exercises. Remember to exercise at the level that is most comfortable for you.
- Open the channels of vital energy in your body and keep them open. Feel your power and energy flowing through your body.
- Use proper body mechanics when sitting, standing, lifting an object, lying down, and so forth.
- Maintain proper posture. Review the section on proper posture on page 252.
- Don't overdo it. Evidence is mounting that excessive loading with heavy weights can increase the risk for acute lower back traumas, can cause increased back pain, and is harmful to the lower back.
- Work out with a partner, if possible.
- Chart your daily, weekly, and monthly workouts.
- Try to exercise the same time every day.
- Psych yourself up. Put inspiring, encouraging, upbeat stickers and slogans around the house, at work, and in your car.
- Remember, a winner never quits and a quitter never wins. You are a winner! You can do it!

Proper Body Mechanics

Whether you are standing, sitting, lying down, walking, running, bending, lifting, or performing any other type of activity, you should employ the four basic protective mechanisms to avoid back injury:

1. Make sure your back is straight—not hunched or swayed.
2. Tuck your buttocks under and tilt your pelvis forward. This helps flatten the lower back spine and also helps tighten the abdominal muscles.
3. Tighten your stomach muscles. This will help strengthen your abdominal muscles and lend greater support to your lower back. It will also push your internal organs back toward your spine so that they don't protrude, pulling your spine out of alignment.
4. Keep your knees relaxed and slightly bent. This makes it easier to maintain proper posture. By keeping the knees bent, you are helping your legs work as shock absorbers for the spine. This is especially true when lifting, bending, twisting, moving, or carrying heavy objects. Bent knees decrease the physical stress on the spine.

LIFTING TIPS

Knowing and using proper body mechanics when lifting can help prevent back pain. Follow these guidelines:

- When lifting, keep your back straight, your knees bent, and your feet shoulder-width apart.
- As you lift, tip your pelvis forward and tighten your abdominal muscles.
- Keep whatever you are lifting close to your torso. Holding objects at arm's length can place increased stress on your back.
- Don't bend forward or twist when lifting.
- If your activity prohibits you from keeping your spine straight (for example, if you are lifting heavy packages out of a deep car trunk), at least follow the remaining guidelines to prevent back injury.

Proper Permanent Posture

Poor posture places added stress on your spine and disks and results in back and joint pain as well as the premature degeneration of your disks. To help change unhealthy habits and avoid future back problems, be sure to maintain correct posture.

When walking, tip your pelvis slightly forward and pull in your stomach. Make sure your shoulders are back, your head is up, and your chin is not protruding forward. Be sure to wear comfortable low-heeled shoes.

Pillows and supports can help you maintain proper posture. For example, when you are driving long distances or sitting for extended periods of time, place a rolled-up towel or pillow behind the small of your back. Sit in chairs with good lower back support. When sleeping on your back, place a pillow under your knees. If sleeping on your side, try placing a pillow between your knees.

To help encourage proper posture, try this exercise:

- When standing, with knees slightly bent, press your lower back against a wall.
- Roll your midback against the wall, then press your head against the wall.
- Now, walk away from the wall and sustain this posture.

BUSY-AS-A-BEE EXERCISES

Too much to do and too little time! We all feel the stress, the time crunch. So what happens if you feel back pain on the job, at school, or at play and can't get away to exercise? The following exercises can be done on the run throughout the day and can help prevent pain in your back.

Cross-Patterning (Standing Up)
- Standing upright, raise your right arm and left leg.
- Turn your head to the side of the raised arm.
- Bend at the knees.
- Repeat using the left arm and right leg.
- Make movements continuous and flowing from one side to the other.

- Duration: 5 minutes.
- Frequency: on rising, mid-morning, and mid-afternoon, or as needed.

Chair March (Sitting at Your Desk or Kitchen Table) This exercise is like marching in place.

- Squeeze your abdominal muscles.
- Tip your pelvis forward.
- Slowly bring one knee up off the chair (a few inches), then slowly switch to the other leg.
- Hold for 5 counts or more.
- Repeat 8 to 10 times.

When Driving the Car (Sitting)
- Tighten your abdominal muscles.
- Tip your pelvis forward.
- Roll/bend shoulders slightly forward until you feel a comfortable stretch in your back.
- Keep your eyes on the road.
- Hold for 30 counts or more.
- Repeat 8 to 10 times.

Sitting (on a Bench, at a Desk, or at the Kitchen Table)
This exercise relaxes back muscles and stretches the lower back.

- Sit on your chair.
- Tilt your pelvis forward.
- Inhale through the mouth, then exhale slowly as you bend forward.
- Bend forward from the hips.
- Let your chest rest on your legs (if you can) or as far forward as possible.
- Let your head and arms drop forward in a relaxed position.
- Hold and relax for up to 30 counts.
- Return to a sitting upright position: Begin with the tailbone, then lower back, midback, shoulders, back, neck, and head.

Wall Exercise (Standing) This exercise relaxes and stretches back muscles, strengthens abdominal muscles, and helps flatten a hyperaccentuated lower back curve.

- Stand with your back against the wall.
- Tip your pelvis forward.
- Squeeze your buttocks.
- Tighten your abdominal muscles.
- Slowly move your feet forward to 1 foot from the wall while sliding your back down the wall.
- Hold as long as you can (5 to 60 counts).
- Repeat as needed.

Back Rest (Lying)

- Lie on your back.
- Flatten your back on the floor.
- Put your legs on a chair or stool.
- Place a pillow under your tailbone.
- Put your arms at your sides or clasp your hands (relaxed) on your stomach.
- Hold this position for 10 to 15 minutes.
- Breathe easily, in through your nose and out through the mouth (see breathing section in this book).
- Meditate. This is an excellent position in which to meditate.

"Chair" Workstation Exercises (Sitting)

- Use good posture wherever you work.
- Keep your head upright with your neck and shoulders relaxed.
- Your forearms should be parallel to the floor with your wrists straight.
- Your lower back should be supported. Fit the backrest snugly against your back.
- Your feet should be flat on the floor or supported by a footrest.
- Frequently change position.

RAPID REVIEW

To prevent future spinal and health problems, you must remember healthy habits.

- Keep a positive mental attitude.
- Meditate daily—sweep your mind clean daily.
- Eat enzyme-rich fresh foods and take nutritional supplements.
- Exercise daily. Perform the exercises in chapter 9, and you'll feel more energy than ever before.
- Use proper body mechanics.
- Maintain proper posture.
- Take time each day to experience newfound energy in your life.
- Never give up! If you miss a day, it's okay. Just get right back on the program.
- Follow this book, and you're going to feel great, look great, and live longer!
- Stick with it!

Conclusion

Conclusion

Regardless of the type or cause of your back pain, you can improve by following the Five-Step Jump-Start Plus Program:

- Keep a positive mental attitude. Regain your emotional balance. Have a positive expectancy. Practice optimism. A positive mental attitude can speed your recovery time (see chapter 7). Hope is a mental muscle, so develop and strengthen it. Be like water—give, adapt, be flexible. The great oceans of the world show us the power of water as well as its adaptability! Be like water.
- Improve your nutritional status as described in chapter 8 by detoxifying regularly; eating right, improving your diet, and following the Five-Step Jump-Start Plus Program's Dietary Do's and Don'ts; and taking supplemental vitamins, minerals, enzymes, and herbs.
- Strengthen the body through the exercises in chapter 9. Exercising can improve circulation to the damaged area, remove toxins, increase flexibility of the surrounding muscles, and increase range of motion. The additional techniques described in chapter 8 can help return you to health and relieve your back pain.
- Develop better habits of time management.
- Rest; take time to rest and get plenty of sleep.
- Count your blessings (instead of sheep) each and every day. Make a habit of being thankful.
- Simplify your life.
- Forgiveness is golden! Life is too short to hold a grudge. Get rid of the garbage. Garbage is for the garbage man. Who needs to carry it around?
- Remember to consult a physician immediately in the event of a serious injury. Signs of a serious injury include severe pain, loss of function, an injury to a joint, or pain that does not resolve within two weeks.

As you can see, this book is a back pain bible and is essential for you and yours. As you review the book daily, you will grow in confidence. Combining successful Eastern and Western philosophies and therapies for the body, mind, and spirit can help you live a longer, happier, pain-free life. Included in these philosophies is that of Traditional Chinese Medicine. The Chinese believe that health is the result of harmony with nature, both in our body and in the environment around us. Harmony is an extension of balancing complementary opposites—that is, yin and yang.

The Five-Step Jump-Start Plus Program succeeded in rehabilitating my son David plus thousands of patients, and brings to you the findings of the ancient healers along with the research of modern science. Pick and choose from the chapters on emotional harmony (chapter 7), nutritional power (chapter 8), and physical healing secrets (chapter 9). Repeat the Five-Step Jump-Start Plus Program on a daily basis. Be consistent.

We know that most people are not emotionally, nutritionally, or physically fit. Being physically fit is important, but being emotionally and nutritionally fit is also critical.

To succeed, you must be honest with yourself and have a strategy. The following points will help you develop a winning program—a winning strategy.

- Believe that you can do it. Repeat to yourself, "I can do it. I know I can do it."
- Set personal goals and put them into action! Write down your goals and review them daily. Setting and reaching goals will give you a sense of purpose.
- Exercise and meditate daily.
  - Exercise thirty minutes every day (four to five times per week at a minimum). If you miss a day, get right back on the program the next day.
  - Meditate daily. Get still. Bring it together and focus—center.
  - Learn and practice relaxation techniques. Have fun! Play! Recharge your body, mind, and soul.

- Laugh and smile more. See the sunny, funny side of life. Lighten your emotional load with humor.

- Consistency is the key to success. Have a program and take each day as it comes, one day at a time. Try to exercise, eat, and meditate the same time every day. This will help you to internalize the program and help make it a daily habit. If you miss a workout or a meditation session one day, start right back on the program the next day.

- Continually psyche yourself up to stick with the program. Remember, what the mind conceives, the body achieves! Put little "upper" phrases wherever you can—in your bedroom, bathroom, kitchen, in books, over the television, in your car—wherever possible.

- Chart your progress. Make or buy a chart showing days, months, and the year or buy a twelve-month pocket planner. Preplan each day and check off times for meditation, exercise, supplements, and eating. Office supply stores carry charts showing the year at a glance with boxes for each day. This type of chart is good for me and keeps me honest. It is also a great reinforcer, because as you check off the meditation, exercise, and nutrition for each day, you can visually see your progress and your accomplishments. You can even write down the number of minutes you exercise each day. This is what my son David did once he was old enough to write.

- Use the buddy system. If possible, work out with a buddy—a friend, wife, husband, or significant other. If no other buddy is available, be your own buddy. You are a special person and you're worth it!

- Internalize my Five-Step Jump-Start Plus Program. Repeat it daily, weekly, monthly, yearly. Be like the little train that could. Repeatedly say to yourself, "I know I can, I know I can," and you can!

- Each and every day, reach for the sky and grab a handful of stars!

Appendix A

BACK PAIN SPECIALISTS

At least 80 percent of people suffering from back pain will recover using the information in this book. However, if your back pain does not resolve, then you should see a doctor or therapist.

There are a number of health care professionals who make the care of back problems one of their main treatment thrusts. There are chiropractors, naturopaths, orthopedists, osteopaths, neurologists, physical therapists, acupuncturists, and massage therapists.

So how do you decide what type of specialist to see if you're suffering from back pain? My training is in chiropractic medicine, so of course I am a little biased. But I believe that any individual with back pain should first be seen by a chiropractor, naturopath, or other conservative back pain specialist. This practitioner will examine you, evaluate the status of your back condition, and develop a treatment program for you to follow. Many physicians may refer you to any number of therapists for adjunctive care. For instance, a massage therapist can help relax tense back muscles and other soft tissue, while a physical therapist may help relieve pain by using electrical stimulation, massage, traction, or other noninvasive techniques. Nutritional consultants give ongoing dietary advice. A licensed acupuncturist will use acupuncture to break up any obstructions and stimulate the flow of chi. However, in many chiropractic and naturopathic offices, all of these services are available, as well as acupressure and other Traditional Chinese Medicine treatments.

Your general medical practitioner may be a wonderful person. However, chances are that he or she has little training in back problems. When back pain strikes, seek the services of a well-trained back specialist. Let this specialist help you through the quagmire and out of the confusion.

If your case involves a fracture, herniation, or other more serious condition, your physician will refer you to an orthopedist (bone specialist) or even to a neurologist or a neurosurgeon (nerve specialists). These specialists, usually seen by referral only, may choose drugs, surgery, or other invasive techniques to treat your back problem.

CHIROPRACTORS

Chiropractic medicine is the largest conservative health care profession in the world. Conservative therapy does not use drugs or surgery in helping the body to help itself. Chiropractors are neuromusculoskeletal specialists. In addition to spinal manipulation, many chiropractors use nutrition, diet, and supplement counseling (advice on natural supplements such as enzymes, minerals, vitamins, herbs, functional foods, and homeopathy), physiotherapy (including electrical stimulation, ultrasound, hydrotherapy, traction, trigger-point therapy, acupuncture, acupressure, ice, transcutaneous electronic nerve stimulation [TENS], heat, diathermy, superficial and deep muscle massage, shiat-su, reflexology, ear acupuncture [staple puncture], and arch and back supports), and therapeutic exercises.

In 1980, I conducted a study with Dr. Brian Bergemann (with the cooperation of the medical director from the Oregon Workers' Compensation Division) to measure the cost-effectiveness of medical versus chiropractic treatment of lower back strains and sprains. We reviewed the insurance files of 227 patients ranging in age from sixteen to sixty-seven years. We found that those treated by chiropractic physicians returned to work faster and at a lower cost to the insurance company than those treated by other methods.

Choosing a Chiropractor

Just as there are individual treatment differences in various healing arts professions, so are there individual differences in the treatment of patients within the chiropractic profession.

How do you choose the chiropractor best suited for you? Seeing a chiropractor will probably be a more personal "hands-on" experience than you've ever had with any other doctor.

In choosing a chiropractor, it is important to discover the doctor's approach to his or her profession. Question potential chiropractors about their techniques and philosophy. Although licensed doctors of chiropractic are well trained and have passed licensing boards, their philosophies of practice may vary slightly. Those who use a holistic approach—including manual adjustments, nutritional counseling or therapy (vitamins, minerals, enzymes, and herbs), physiological therapy (including acupressure, massage, electrical stimulation, traction, ice, and heat), and applied kinesiology—are called "mixers." Then there are the "straight" chiropractors; they do not usually use adjunctive therapy but emphasize removal of spinal nerve interference by hands only. However, both approaches can relieve back pain, and all chiropractors emphasize preventive chiropractic care, correction of vertebral misalignments or subluxations, and nerve function restoration.

A little homework in choosing a chiropractor might be helpful.

1. Talk to friends. How do they like their chiropractors?
2. Call your national, state, or local chiropractic associations.
3. Read books on chiropractic, especially my book *Introduction to Chiropractic Health.*[1]

For information on chiropractic, an extensive bibliography, or additional studies on the health benefits of chiropractic, contact:

The American Chiropractic Association
1701 Clarendon Boulevard
Arlington, VA 22209
Tel: 1-800-986-4636
Fax: (703) 243-2593
Internet: http://www.amerchiro.org

or

International Chiropractors Association
1110 North Glebe Road, Suite 1000
Arlington, VA 22201
Tel: 1-800-423-4690 or (703) 528-5000
Fax: (703) 528-5023
Internet: www.chiropractic.org

NATUROPATHS

Naturopathy (or "natural cure") is a concept of healing that uses a wide variety of therapies, including lifestyle modification, homeopathy, physiotherapy, nutrition, botanical medicine, acupuncture, hydrotherapy, counseling, and many other natural techniques. In addition, many naturopaths practice chiropractic techniques as well. Naturopathy is a profession that is exploding in popularity. For more information on naturopathy, contact:

The American Association of Naturopathic Physicians
601 Valley Street, Suite 105
Seattle, WA 98109
Tel: (206) 298-0125
Internet: http://naturopathic.org/

NEUROLOGISTS

Neurologists are medical doctors who specialize in the diagnosis and treatment of conditions affecting the nervous system. Because the nervous system sends messages of pain and is directly involved in most serious back conditions, a neurologist's examination and consultation can be very important for any condition that involves the nerves. A neurologist usually works closely with your treating physician. For more information, contact:

The American Neurological Association
5841 Cedar Lake Road, Suite 108
Minneapolis, MN 55416
Tel: (612) 545-6284

ORTHOPEDISTS

Orthopedists are medical doctors trained to treat the musculoskeletal system, including the bones, joints, muscles, ligaments, and tendons. The orthopedist mainly uses drugs and surgery to treat back pain. Orthopedists may refer patients to chiropractors for adjustment and therapy or to physical therapists or other specialists. For more information about orthopedists, contact:

The American Academy of Orthopaedic Surgeons
6300 North River Road
Rosemont, IL 60018-4262
Tel: 1-800-346-2267
Internet: http://www.aaos.org/

OSTEOPATHS

Doctors of Osteopathy are trained to treat disorders and diseases with special emphasis on the musculoskeletal system. Strengthening the immune system is an important part of their treatment. For more information about osteopaths, contact:

The American Osteopathic Association
142 East Ontario Street
Chicago, IL 60611
Tel: 1-800-621-1773
Fax: (312) 202-8200
Internet: http://www.am-osteo-assn.org/

PHYSICAL THERAPISTS

Physical therapists (PTs) are health care professionals who evaluate and treat individuals suffering from injuries or disease. Their treatment may include therapeutic exercise, massage, ultrasound, transcutaneous nerve stimulation (TNS), cardiovascular endurance training, and training in activities of daily living. Physical therapists usually require referral from a physician and work in conjunction with orthopedists, neurosurgeons, and other specialists. For more information about physical therapists, contact:

The American Physical Therapy Association
1111 North Fairfax Street
Alexandria, VA 22314-1488
Tel: (703) 684-APTA
Fax: (703) 684-7343
Internet: http://www.apta.org/public_relations/ptfact.htm

ACUPUNCTURISTS

Acupuncturists are health care providers licensed to practice acupuncture and are usually used as adjunctive therapy in conjunction with other primary therapies.

Acupuncture is a therapy that uses very thin steel needles inserted painlessly into nerve endings or points of vital energy along meridians of the body. In so doing, vital organs, the brain, and the nervous system are stimulated.

An acupuncturist can treat over 250 conditions and ailments. This includes back-related disorders such as arthritis, bursitis, cramps, headaches, neuralgia, neuritis, sciatica, sprains, strains, and stress, as well as other conditions ranging from asthma to facial paralysis, stroke, or ringing in the ears (tinnitus). Acupuncture is also used as an anesthetic during operations and to relieve postoperative pain. Further, acupuncture has been effective in treating alcohol, tobacco, and drug addiction.

How does acupuncture work? Chinese neurological researchers have found that acupuncture stimulates the brain. The brain then releases enkephalins and endorphins (two neuropeptides). These substances act like morphine and cause the anesthetic action to take place.

In addition, nerve transmission apparently can be blocked using acupuncture needles on the specific meridian, resulting in a form of anesthesia. Through acupuncture, the messages of pain are blocked from reaching the brain, thus decreasing or eliminating perceived pain.

Finally, Chinese physicians feel that when acupuncture needles are placed on specific meridians, there is stimulation of the vital organ to which the meridian is connected. Stimulating the vital organ helps to bring the organ into harmony with the body and allows the organ to better cope with any illness that might be attacking it. For example, to treat chronic back pain, one would needle the kidney and liver meridians with possible spleen and heart involvement.

It should be noted that acupuncturists undergo extensive training to perfect their technique. Further, although acupressure can be self-administered in using certain easily accessible points for treating specific conditions and diseases, complete acupressure treatment, acupuncture, or moxibustion requires professional care and advice. Finally, acupuncture, acupressure, moxibustion, and herbal medicine should be used simultaneously to correct any imbalance and to decrease and eliminate the underlying cause of back pain.

Acupuncture and acupressure are also used as adjunctive therapy with surgery to control pain.

For more information, contact:

American Association of Acupuncture and Bio-Energetic Medicine
2512 Manoa Road
Honolulu, HI 96822
Tel: (808) 926-2069
Fax: (808) 946-0378
Internet: http://www.healthy.net/aaabem/

THE RISE OF ALTERNATIVE HEALTH CARE

The use of alternative health care is skyrocketing in both consumer popularity and government acceptance: "Based on peer-reviewed studies, as many as 60 million adults are using alternative medicine therapies in conjunction with conventional medical treatments for various health-related concerns. According to a recent national study of alternative medicine and its use among adults in the United States. . . . 40 percent of all survey respondents reported using some form of alternative health care in the year prior to participating in the mail survey."[2]

Recognizing the limits of conventional medicine, particularly in treating chronic illnesses and back pain, consumers are looking for options. According to a front-page story by Erin Hoover Barnett in *The Oregonian*,[3] exciting new programs bring a new meaning to life and health both in the Northwest and in the nation. Consider the following:

- Nature's Fresh Northwest, a grocery chain with organic produce and health foods, opened a Lake Oswego, Oregon store in August 1998, with a pharmacy for prescription drugs combined with an herbal supplement dispensary. Customers can consult with a naturopath and/or pharmacist and look up herbs and medications on an online computer network or read about them in a library and bookstore above the pharmacy. Also, consumers can take yoga classes or soak in a German hydrotherapy tub.
- The Oregon Health Sciences University (OHSU) medical school will inaugurate an annual lecture on alternative medicine, adding to coursework already offered.
- Kaiser Permanente plans to offer limited coverage for acupuncture and naturopathic medicine. Kaiser already covers chiropractic care, as do most other big health insurers.
- The Oregon Cancer Center at OHSU is starting research on alternative therapies for cancer.
- Wild Oats Market Inc. tentatively plans to launch as many as ten alternative "wellness" stores in the Northwest. A national roll-out is on the horizon, if the concept catches on. Using this format, naturopaths, chiropractors, druggists, and others will work together, giving classes and consultation in yoga (and other exercises), meditation, postive thinking, and nutrition.[4]

Appendix B

MANUFACTURERS AND DISTRIBUTORS OF BACK CARE PRODUCTS

Anabolic Labs
P.O. Box C19508
Irvine, CA 92713
Tel: (714) 863-0340
Fax: (714) 261-2928

Distributes Anabolic Foot Orthotics, special devices worn in your shoes to stabilize your feet and help maintain spinal alignment, improve posture, and help eliminate a key cause of back problems.

Back Technologies, Inc.
2525 West Casino Road
Everett, WA 98204
Tel: (206) 355 5900 or
1-800-643-2225

Manufactures and distributes The Back Machine and other quality back relief products.

Bodyline Comfort Systems
3730 Kori Road
Jacksonville, FL 32257
Tel: (904) 262-4068
Fax: (904) 262-2225

Distributes lumbar support cushions; cervical support pillows; a contoured mattress overlay; ankle and knee braces; and traction units, among other products.

Cequal Products
1328 Sixteenth Street
Santa Monica, CA 90404
Tel: (310) 394-1113 or
1-800-350-2998
Fax: (310) 395-3218

Distributes cold packs, backrests (compact/self-inflating), footstools, reading stands, and The Swezey Institute video- and audiotapes.

Crescent Products
7410 Lakeland Avenue North
Minneapolis, MN 55428
Tel: 1-800-989-8085

Offers the Crescent Memory Pillow.

Enrichments
P.O. Box 579
Hinsdale, IL 60521
Tel: 1-800-323-5547

Offers long-handled shoehorns, long-handled reacher, and other back relief and assistive products.

Ever-Flex, Inc.
1656 John A. Papalas Drive
Lincoln Park, MI 48146
Tel: 1-800-877-2844

Offers orthotics and foam insoles.

Fitness to Go
P.O. Box 266
Independence, MO 64051
Tel: 1-800-821-3126

Manufactures and distributes Mini-Gym isokinetic exercisers.

Foot Levelers, Inc.
518 Pocahontas Avenue, NE
P. O. Box 12611
Roanoke, VA 24027-2611
Tel: 1-800-553-4860 (USA)
Tel: 1-800-344-4860 (Canada)
Fax: (540) 345-0202

Distributes custom-made foot orthotics.

Hoyle Products
302 Orange Grove
Fillmore, CA 93015-1938
Tel: (805) 524-1211 or
1-800-345-1950

Offers lap desks for reading in bed.

LBM, Inc.
P.O. Box 3911
Chesterfield, MO 63006
Tel: 1-800-325-1153

Offers heel lifts, orthopedic supports, and herbal products.

Life Fitness
10601 West Belmont Avenue
Franklin Park, IL 60131
Tel: 1-800-735 8367 or
(847) 288 3300

Manufactures the Lifecycle Exercise Bike and a variety of fitness machines for health clubs and homes.

McCarty's
3329 Industrial Avenue
Coeur d'Alene, ID 83814
Tel: 1-800-635-3557

Manufactures Sacro-Ease line of portable backrest support products for car seats and other uses.

MDC
8580 Milliken Avenue
Rancho Cucamonga, CA 91730
Tel: 1-800-472-4221

Offers magnet massage devices.

Mediflow
Unit #11,
130 Konrad Crescent
Markham, Ontario
L3R 065 Canada
Tel: 1-800-308 3069

Offers waterbase cervical pillows.

Nikken U.S.A., Inc.
15363 Barranca Parkway
Irvine, CA 92718
Tel: (949) 789-2000
Fax: (949) 789-2080

Offeres magnetic products, nutritional supplements, numerous supports, and other products.

NordicTrack
104 Peavey Road
Chaska, MN 55318
Tel: 1-800-328-5888

Manufactures and distributes the NordicTrack line of fitness products.

OMS Medical Supplies
1950 Washington Street
Braintree, MA 02184
Tel: 1-800-323-1839

Offers acupuncture needles, biomagnets, and supports.

Performance Health, Inc.
127 Craighead Street, Suite 105
Pittsburgh, PA 15211
Tel: 1-800-BIOFREEZE

Offers Biofreeze, a pain-relieving gel.

The Pillow Place
1940 Moores Mill Road, NW
Atlanta, GA 30318
Tel: 1-800-832-2022

Offers cervical pillows and lumbar wedges and pillows.

Pleasing Patients Unlimited
221 North Robertson
Boulevard, #C-1
Beverly Hills, CA 90211
Tel: 1-800-521-5672

Offers neck pillows, magnets, and other products.

PTmart, Inc.
5412 South Mingo Road, #K
Tulsa, OK 74146
Tel: 1-800-331-3829

Offers the PTball.

Relax the Back Store
15660 SW Pacific, Suite A3
Tigard, OR 97224
Tel: (503) 684-8494
or call 1-800-290-2225
for a store near you.

Offers an extensive array of lifestyle products designed to automatically correct your posture and relieve pain.

Synergy Therapeutic Systems
620 Douglas Avenue, Suite 1308
Altamonte Springs, FL 32714
Tel: 1-800-639-3539
Fax: (407) 786-2646

Offers thoracic and cervical kits containing exercise instructions and devices.

Tempur-Pedic
848G Nandino Boulevard
Lexington, KY 40511
Tel: 1-800-878-8889

Offers pillows, supports, and pressure relief products.

Tools for Exploration
4460 Redwood Highway, Suite 2
San Rafael, CA 94903
Tel: (415) 499-9050 or
1-800-456-9887
Fax: (415) 499-9047

Suppliers of a wide range of magnetic products.

Topper Sportsmedicine
5808 South Rapp Street, Suite 109
Littleton, CO 80120
Tel: 1-800-250-3779
Fax: (303) 791-2254

Offers The Original Sport Cord for rehabilitative exercise.

Appendix C

COMPANIES THAT MANUFACTURE OR DISTRIBUTE NUTRITIONAL PRODUCTS TO HELP YOUR BACK

A.C. Grace Company
1100 Quitman Road
P.O. Box 570
Big Sandy, TX 75777
Tel: 1-800-833-4368

Advanced Medical Nutrition, Inc.
2247 National Avenue
Hayward, CA 04545
Tel: 1-800-437-8888
Fax: (510) 783-8196

AK Pharma Inc.
P.O. Box 111
Pleasantville, NJ 08232
Tel: 1-800-257-8650
Fax: (201) 432-6183

American Biologics
1180 Walnut Avenue
Chula Vista, CA 91911
Tel: 1-800-227-4458
Fax: (619) 429-8004

American Health
90 Orville Drive
Bohemia, NY 11716
Tel: 1-800-345-4152 or
(516) 244-2021
Fax: (516) 244-1777

American Image Marketing
3904 East Flamingo Avenue
Nampa, ID 83687
Tel: 1-800-477-4246

American Laboratories, Inc.
4410 South 102nd Street
Omaha, NE 68127
Tel: (402) 339-2494 or
1-800-445-5985
Fax: (402) 339-0801

Anabolic Laboratories
17801 Gillette Avenue
P.O. Box C19508
Irvine, CA 92713
Tel: (714) 863-0340
Fax: (714) 261-2928

Arise & Shine
3225 North Los Altos Avenue
Tucson, AZ 85718
Tel: (602) 293-1098
Fax: (602) 887-1244

BioDynamax
6525 Gunpark Drive, #150–507
Boulder, CO 80301-3338
Tel: (303) 530-4665 or
1-800-926-7525
Fax: (303) 516-5234

Bioenergy Nutrients
6565 Odell Place
Boulder, CO 80301-3330
Tel: 1-800-627-7775
Fax: (303) 530-2592

Biogenetics Food Corporation
4475 Corporate Square
Naples, FL 33942
Tel: 1-800-926-5100
Fax: (941) 592-9338

Bio-Health
22865 Lake Forest Drive
Lake Forest, CA 92630
Tel: 1-800-500-4610

Biotec Foods
1 Capitol District
250 South Hotel Street, Suite 200
Honolulu, HI 96813
Tel: 1-800-331-5888
Fax: 1-800-788-1083

Biotics Research Corporation
P.O. Box 36888
Houston, TX 77236
Tel: 1-800-231-5777
Fax: (281) 344-0725

Body Mechanics
624 Estuary Drive
Bradenton, FL 34209
Tel: 1-800-264-1114

Botanical Laboratories, Inc.
1441 West Smith Road
Bellingham, WA 98226
Tel: (360) 384-5656
Fax: (360) 384-1140

Christmas Natural Foods Ltd.
#203-8173 128th Street
Surrey, BC
V3W 4G1 Canada
Tel: (604) 591-8881 or
1-800-663-6559
Fax: 1-800-661-6559

Colema Boards, Inc.
P.O. Box 229
Anderson, CA 96007
Tel: (916) 365-2496
Fax: (916) 347-5921

Dee Cee Laboratories, Inc.
304 Dee Cee Court
P.O. Box 383
White House, TN 37188
Tel: 1-800-251-8182
Fax: (615) 672-4489

Douglas Laboratories
6000 Boyce Road
Pittsburgh, PA 15205
Tel: 1-888-DOUGLAB
Fax: 1-888-245-4440

Dr. Enzyme Health Products
P.O. Box 92094
Portland, OR 97292-2094
Tel: (503) 256-9901
Fax: (503) 256-1730

Elite Health Foods & Products
2881 Green Valley Parkway
Henderson, NV 89014
Tel: 1-800-722-8181
Fax: (702) 877-9172

Emerson Ecologics
18 Lomar Park
Pepperell, MA 01463-1416
Tel: 1-800-654-4432
Fax: 1-800-718-7238

Enzymatic Therapy, Inc.
825 Challenger Drive
Green Bay, WI 54311
Tel: 1-800-558-7372 or
(414) 469-1313
Fax: (414) 469-4400
http://www.enz.com

Enzyme Process Laboratories
2035 East Cedar Street
Tempe, AZ 85281
Tel: 1-800-521-8669
Fax: (602) 731-9432

Garden State Nutritionals
8 Henderson Drive
West Caldwell, NJ 07006
Tel: 1-800-526-9095
Fax: (973) 276-7111

General Nutrition Centers
Customer Service
921 Penn Avenue
Pittsburgh, PA 15222
Tel: 1-800-477-4462

General Research Laboratories
8900 Winnetka Avenue
Northridge, CA 91324
Tel: 1-800-421-1856
Fax: (818) 407-8500

Genuine Enzymes
8500 NW River Park Drive, #223
Parkville, MO 64152
Tel: 1-800-637-7893
Fax: (816) 746-8387

Green Foods Corporation
320 North Graves Avenue
Oxnard, CA 93030
Tel: 1-800-777-4430
Fax: (805) 983-8843

Health Care Technologies, Ltd.
P.O. Box 528
Broomfield, CA 80038-0528

Health Now
387 Ivy Street
San Francisco, CA 94102

Health Smart Vitamins
Attn: Customer Service Department
1921 Miller Drive
Longmont, CO 80501
Tel: 1-800-492-3003
Fax: (303) 530-2592

Hyssop® Enterprises
7095 Hollywood Boulevard, Suite 713
Hollywood, CA 90028

InterHealth Nutraceuticals Inc.
1320 Galaxy Way
Concord, CA 94520
Tel: (925) 827-4400 or
1-800-783-4636
Fax: (925) 827-4088

International Enzyme Foundation, Inc.
P.O. Box 249, Highway 160
Forsyth, MO 65653
Tel: 1-800-433-8589
Fax: (816) 746-8382

International Nutrition, Inc.
6185 Harrison Drive, Suite 1
Las Vegas, NV 89120
Tel: 1-800-535-6442

J.R. Carlson Laboratories, Inc.
15 College
Arlington Heights, IL 60004
Tel: 1-800-323-4141
Fax: (847) 255-1605

Kyolic, Ltd.
23501 Madero
Mission Viejo, CA 92691
Tel: 1-800-527-5200
Fax: (949) 958-2764

Lane Labs
110 Commerce Drive
Allendale, NJ 07401
Tel: 1-800-526-3005
Fax: (201) 236-9091

Maitake Products, Inc.
P.O. Box 1354
Paramus, NJ 07653
Tel: 1-800-747-7418
Fax: (201) 229-0585

Malabar Formulas
28537 Nuevo Valley Drive
Nuevo, CA 92567
Tel: 1-800-426-6617
Fax: (909) 928-4038

Marcor Development
108 John Street
Hackensack, NJ 07601
Tel: (201) 489-5700
Fax: (201) 489-7357

McNeil Consumer Products Co.
7050 Camp Hill Road
Ft. Washington, PA 19034
Tel: 1-800-522-8243
Fax: (215) 273-4070

Miller Pharmacal Group, Inc.
4562 Prime Parkway
McHenry, IL 60050
Tel: 1-800-323-2935
Fax: (630) 871-9558

M.M.S. (Murdock Pharmaceutical)
10 Mountain Spring Parkway
Springville, UT 84663
Tel: 1-800-962-8873
Fax: (801) 489-1640

Modern Products, Inc.
3015 West Vera Avenue
Milwaukee, WI 53209
Tel: (414) 352-3333
Fax: (414) 242-2751

Mucos Pharma GmbH & Co.
Alpenstrasse 29
D-8192 Geretsried 1 Germany
Tel: (+49) 0-8171-5180
Fax: (+49) 0-8171-52008

Natren, Inc.
3105 Willow Lane
Westlake Village, CA 91361
Tel: 1-800-992-3323
Fax: (805) 371-4742

Natrol, Inc.
20731 Marilla Street
Chatsworth, CA 91311
Tel: 1-800-326-1520
Fax: (818) 739-6001

Natural Balance or Pep Products, Inc.
3130 North Commerce Court
P.O. Box 715
Castle Rock, CO 80104
Tel: 1-800-624-4260
Fax: (303) 688-1591

Natural Life
10 Mountain Spring Parkway
Springville, UT 84663
Tel: 1-800-531-3233
Fax: 1-800-489-3302

Naturally Vitamin Supplements Co.
14851 North Scottsdale Road
Scottsdale, AZ 85254
Tel: 1-800-899-4499
Fax: (602) 991-0551

Nature's Plus
10 Daniel Street
Farmingdale, NY 11735
Tel: 1-800-645-9500
Fax: 1-888-665-0628

Nature's Sunshine Products, Inc.
P.O. Box 19005
Provo, UT 84605-9005
Tel: (801) 342-4300
Fax: (801) 342-4305

Nature's Way Products, Inc.
10 Mountain Springs Parkway
Springville, UT 84663
Tel: (801) 489-3639
Fax: (801) 489-1640

New Spirit Naturals, Inc.
458 West Arrow Highway, Suite C
San Dumas, CA 91733
Tel: 1-800-922-2766
Fax: (909) 599-4035

NF Formulas, Inc.
805 SE Sherman
Portland, OR 97214-4666
Tel: 1-800-547-4891
Fax: (503) 682-9529

NOW Natural Foods
550 Mitchell Avenue
Glendale Heights, IL 60139
Tel: 1-800-999-8069
Fax: 1-800-886-1045

Nutraceutical Corp.
(also Solaray, Premier One, Veg Life, Natural Max, Solar Green, Natural Sport, and Trout Lake Farms)
2815 Industrial Drive
Ogden, UT 84401
Tel: 1-800-579-4665 or
1-800-669-8877
Fax: (801) 621-2961

Nutrissential Corporation
1902 East Meadowmere
Springfield, MO 65804
Tel: 1-800-637-7893
Fax: (816) 746-8387

Nutrition 21
1010 Turquoise Street, Suite 335
San Diego, CA 92109
Tel: 1-800-343-3082
Fax: (619) 488-7316

Nutritional Enzyme Support System (NESS)
8500 NW River Park Drive, #223
Parkville, MO 64152
Tel: 1-800-637-7893
Fax: (816) 746-8387

Nutri-West/NutriQuest
P.O. Box 950
Douglas, WY 82633
Tel: (307) 358-5066 or
1-800-443-3333
Fax: (307) 358-9208

PhysioLogics
6565 Odell Place
Boulder, CO 80301-3330
Tel: 1-800-765-6775 or
(303) 530-4554
Fax: (303) 530-2592 or
(303) 516-5234

Prevail Corporation
2204-8 NW Birdsdale
Gresham, OR 97030
Tel: 1-800-248-0885
Fax: (503) 667-4790

Progena
2501 Baylor SE
Albuquerque, NM 87106

Pro-Pac Labs
3804 Airport Road
Ogden, UT 84405
Tel: (801) 621-0900
Fax: (801) 621-0930

Pure-Gar Inc.
23 Golden Glen
Irvine, CA 92714
Tel: 1-800-822-7701
Fax: (818) 739-6045

Rhema Industries, Ltd.
110-3738 North Fraser Way
Burnaby, BC
V5J 5G1 Canada
Tel: (604) 430-5211

Royal Sun
800 Leilani Street
Hilo, HI 96720
Tel: (808) 969-6747
Fax: (808) 935-1585

Schiff Products, Inc., or Weider Nutrition, International
1960 South 4250 West
Salt Lake City, UT 84104
Tel: (801) 972-0300
Fax: (801) 975-7185

Shinko American Inc.
1450 Broadway
New York, NY 10018
Tel: (212) 398-0550
Fax: (212) 398-9726

Solgar Vitamin and Herb Co.
500 Willow Tree Road
Leonia, NJ 07605
Tel: 1-800-645-2246
Fax: (201) 944-7351

Standard Process
12521 131st Court, NE
Kirkland, WA 98083-2484
Tel: 1-800-292-6699 or
1-800-848-5061
Fax: (877) 821-3179

Sundown-Rexall
851 Broken Sound Parkway, NW
Boca Raton, FL 33487
Tel: 1-800-255-7399
Fax: (561) 995-6881

Thompson Nutritional Products
4031 NE 12th Terrace
Ft. Lauderdale, FL 33334
Tel: 1-800-421-1192
Fax: (561) 995-6883

Titan Laboratories
350 Fifth Avenue, Suite 3304
New York, NY 10118
Tel: 1-800-929-0945
Fax: (352) 628-3444

Triarco
6 Morris Street
Paterson, NJ 07501
Tel: (973) 278-7300
Fax: (973) 942-8873

Twin Laboratories, Inc.
2120 Smithtown Avenue
Ronkonkoma, NY 11779
Tel: (516) 467-3140
Fax: (516) 467-3083

Viobin Corporation
700 East Main Street
P.O. Box 158
Waunakee, WI 53597
Tel: (608) 849-5944

Vitatech International, Inc.
28332 Dow Avenue
Tustin, CA 92680
Tel: (714) 832-9700
Fax: (714) 731-8482

Vitech America Corporation
22703 72nd Avenue South
Kent, WA 98032
Tel: (253) 872-7525
Fax: (253) 859-5912

Wakunaga of America Co., Ltd.
23501 Madero
Mission Viejo, CA 92691
Tel: 1-800-421-2998
Fax: (949) 458-2764

Weider Food Companies
1911 South 3850 West
Salt Lake City, UT 84104
Tel: (801) 972-0300
Fax: (801) 975-7185

Yellow Emperor, Inc.
P.O. Box 2631
Eugene, OR 97402
Tel: (541) 485-6664

Y.H. Products Corporation
400 North Lombard Street
Oxnard, CA 93030
Tel: (805) 983-1130
Fax: (805) 983-3648

Yves Veggie Cuisine
1138 East Georgia
Vancouver, BC
V6A 2AB Canada
Tel: (604) 525-1345
Fax: (604) 525-2555

Zand Herbal Formula
P.O. Box 5312
Santa Monica, CA 90409
Tel: (310) 822-0500
Fax: (310) 822-1050

Notes

ONE

1. J. L. Kelsey and A. A. White, "Epidemiology and Impact of Low Back Pain," *Spine* 5, no. 2 (March 1980): 133–42.

2. C. Leboeuf-Yde and K. O. Kyvik, "At What Age Does Low Back Pain Become a Common Problem? A Study of 29,424 Individuals Aged 12–41 Years," *Spine* 23, no. 2 (January 1998): 228–34.

3. G. B. J. Andersson, "The Epidemiology of Spinal Disorders," in *The Adult Spine: Principles and Practice*, ed. J. W. Frymoyer (New York: Raven Press, 1991), 107–46.

4. B. Vällfors, "Acute, Subacute, and Chronic Low Back Pain: Clinical Symptoms, Absenteeism and Working Environment," *Scandinavian Journal of Rehabilitory Medicine and Supplies* 11 (1985): 1–98.

5. R. A. Sternbach, "Survey of Pain in the United States: The Nuprin Report," *Clinical Journal of Pain* 2, no. 1 (1986): 49–53.

6. R. A. Sternbach, "Pain and 'Hassles' in the United States; Findings of the Nuprin Pain Report," *Pain* 27, no. 1 (October 1986): 69–80.

7. B. K. Cypress, "Characteristics of Physician Visits for Back Symptoms: A National Perspective," *American Journal of Public Health* 73, no. 4 (April 1983): 389–95.

8. L. G. Hart, R. A. Deyo, and D. C. Cherkin, "Physician Office Visits for Low Back Pain: Frequency, Clinical Evaluation, and Treatment Patterns from a U.S. National Survey," *Spine* 20, no. 1 (January 1995): 11–19.

9. Steven J. Linton, "The Socioeconomic Impact of Chronic Back Pain: Is Anyone Benefiting?" *Pain* 75, nos. 2–3 (April 1998): 163–68.

10. L. S. Cunningham and J. L. Kelsey, "Epidemiology of Musculoskeletal Impairments and Associated Disability,"

American Journal of Public Health 74 (1984): 574–79.

11. U.S. Bureau of the Census, *Statistical Abstract of the United States: 1995* (Washington, D.C., 1995), 8.

12. J. L. Kelsey, P. B. Githens, A. A. White, T. R. Holford, S. D. Walter, T. O'Connor, A. M. Ostfeld, U. Weil, W. O. Southwick, and J. A. Calogero, "An Epidemiologic Study of Lifting and Twisting on the Job and Risk for Acute Prolapsed Lumbar Intervertebral Disk," *Journal of Orthopedic Research* 2, no. 1 (1984): 61–66.

TWO

1. Philip Whitfield, ed., *Human Body Explained* (New York: Henry Holt and Co., 1995), 22.

2. Arthur C. Guyton, *Textbook of Medical Physiology*, 8th ed. (Philadelphia: W. B. Saunders, 1991), 67.

THREE

1. Lao Tze, quoted in *The Tao of Health, Sex, and Longevity*, ed. Daniel Reid (New York: Simon & Schuster, 1989), 8.

FOUR

1. Hans Selye, preface to *The Stress of Life* (New York: McGraw-Hill, 1978).

2. Jeffrey Lotz, "Heavy Lifting Dries Out Vertebral Disks," *Reuters*, 12 June 1998.

3. U.S. Department of Health and Human Services, *The Surgeon General's Report on Nutrition and Health* (Washington, D.C., 1988), 313–18.

4. Rene Caillet, *Neck and Arm Pain* (Philadelphia: FA Davis, 1981).

5. C. H. Willford, C. Kisner T. M. Glenn, and L. Sachs, "The Interaction of Wearing Multifocal Lenses with Head Posture and Pain," *Journal of Orthopedic Sports and Physical Therapy* 23, no. 3 (March 1996): 194–99.

6. National Institutes of Health press release, 17 June 1998.

7. Archibald D. Hart, *Adrenaline and Stress* (Dallas: Word Publishing, 1995), 25.

8. A. Lampe, W. Sollner, M. Kirsmer, G. Rumpold, W. Kantner-Rumplmair, M. Ogon, and G. Rathner, "The Impact of Stressful Life Events on Exacerbation of Chronic Low-Back Pain," *Journal of Psychosomatic Research* 44, no. 5 (May 1998): 555–63.

9. R. A. Sternbach, "Survey of Pain in the United States: The Nuprin Report," *Clinical Journal of Pain* 2, no. 1 (1986): 49–53.

10. R. A. Sternbach, "Pain and 'Hassles' in the United States; Findings of the Nuprin Pain Report," *Pain* 27, no. 1 (October 1986): 69–80.

11. Janet G. Travell and David G. Simons, *Myofascial Pain and Dysfunction* (Baltimore: Williams & Wilkins, 1983).

12. J. B. Cordaro, Testimony to U.S. House of Representatives Committee on Energy and Commerce, Subcommittee on Health and the Environment. Hearing on legislative issues related to the regulation of dietary supplements, 29 July 1993.

FIVE

1. S. Bigos, O. Bowyer, G. Braen, K. Brown, R. Deyo, S. Haldeman, J. Hart, E. Johnson, R. Keller, D. Kido, M. Liang, R. Nelson, M. Nordin, B. Owen, M. Pope, R. Schwartz, D. Stewart, J. Susman, J. Triano, L. Tripp, D. Turk, C. Watts, and J. Weinstein, *Acute Low Back Problems in Adults. Clinical Practice Guideline No. 14*, AHCPR Publication No. 95-0642 (Rockville, Md.: Agency for Health Care Policy and Research, Public Health Service, U.S. Department of Health and Human Services, 1994), 28–34.

2. "A Possible Danger of Cortisone Cream," *Pediatric Report's Child Health Newsletter* 10, no. 2 (1993): 7.

3. S. Bentley, "The Treatment of Sports Injuries by Local Injections," *British Journal of Sports Medicine* 15 (1981): 71–74.

4. B. Zarins, "Soft Tissue Injury and Repair—Biochemical Aspects," *International Journal of Sports Medicine* 3, no. 1 (1982): 9–11.

5. R. B. Traycoff, "Musculoskeletal and Joint Pain," in *Handbook of Chronic Pain Management*, ed. C. D. Tollison (Baltimore: Williams & Wilkins, 1989), 475–89.

6. H. J. Mankin and K. A. Conger, "The Acute Effects of Intra Articular Hydrocortisone on Articular Cartilage in Rabbits," *Journal of Bone and Joint Surgery* 48, A (1966): 1383–88.

7. R. B. Salter, A. Gross, and J. H. Hall, "Hydrocortisone Arthoropathy—An Experimental Investigation," *Canadian Medical Association Journal* 97 (1967): 374–77.

8. E. W. Boland, "Prolonged Uninterrupted Cortisone Therapy in Rheumatoid Arthritis," *British Medical Journal* 2 (1951): 191–99.

9. H. P. Rome and F. J. Braceland, "Psychological Response to Corticotropin, Cortisone and Related Steroid Substances (Psychotic Reaction Types)," *Journal of the American Medical Association* 27 (1952): 148.

10. L. E. Ward, C. H. Slocumb, H. F. Polley, E. W. Lowman, and P. S. Hench, "Clinical Effects of Cortisone Administered Oral to Patients with Rheumatoid Arthritis," *Proceedings of the Staff Meeting at Mayo Clinic* 26 (1951): 361.

11. S. J. Gray, J. A. Benson, Jr., R. W. Reifenstein, and H. M. Spiro, "Chronic Stress and Peptic Ulcer 1. Effect of Corticotropin (ACTH) and Cortisone on Gastric Secretion," *Journal of the American Medical Association* 147 (1951): 1529–84.

12. R. G. Sprague, H. L. Mason, and M. H. Power, *Physiologic Effects of Cortisone and ACTH in Man, Recent Progress in Hormone Research* (New York: Academic Press, 1951).

13. H. Pirga, "Cortisone-Related Glaucoma," (Rumanian)

Oftalmologia 37, no. 2 (1993): 154–56.

14. D. E. Fischer and W. H. Bickel, "Corticosteroid-Induced Avascular Necrosis," *Journal of Bone and Joint Surgery* 53, A (1971): 859–73.

15. M. Pfeiffer and P. Griss, "Schadel-Hirn-Trauma und aseptische Osteonekrose. Steroidbedingte Folgezustande nach Hirnodemtherapie" (Craniocerebral Trauma and Aseptic Osteonecrosis. Steroid-Induced Sequelae after Therapy of Brain Edema), *Unfallchirurg* 95, no. 6 (1992): 284–87.

16. L. H. Chen, S. Liu Cook, M. E. Newell, and K. Barnes, "Survey of Drug Use by the Elderly and Possible Impact of Drugs on Nutritional Status," *Drug Nutrient Interactions* 3 (1985): 73–86.

17. L. E. Rikans, "Drugs and Nutrition in Old Age," *Life Sciences* 39 (1986): 1027–36.

SIX

1. G. Bronfort, "Chiropractic Treatment of Low-Back Pain: A Prospective Survey," *Journal of Manipulative and Physiological Therapy* 9 (1986): 99–113.

2. R. A. Deyo and W. R. Phillips, "Low Back Pain. A Primary Care Challenge," *Spine* 21, 24 (December 1996): 2826–32.

SEVEN

1. Joan C. Priestley, *Your Life Enhancing Diet* (Los Angeles: Center for 21st Century Medicine).

2. Jack Kornfeild, *Four by Alan Watts* (South Burlington, Vt.: Video Collection, 1998), videotape.

3. E. M. Altmaier, D. W. Russell, C. F. Kao, T. R. Lehmann, and J. N. Weinstein, "Role of Self-Efficacy in Rehabilitation Outcome Among Chronic Low Back Pain Patients," *Journal of Counseling Psychology* 40, 3 (1993): 335–39.

4. Daniel P. Reid, *The Tao of Health, Sex, and Longevity* (New York: Simon & Schuster, 1989).

5. C. J. Vander Kolk, R. A. Chubon, and J. K. Vander Kolk, "The Relationship Among Back Injury, Pain, and

Sexual Functioning," *Sexuality and Disability* 10, no. 3 (November 1992): 153–57.

EIGHT

1. Arthur C. Guyton, *Textbook of Medical Physiology*, 8th ed. (Philadelphia: W. B. Saunders, 1991), 274.
2. U.S. House of Representatives Committee on Energy and Commerce, Subcommittee on Health and the Environment. Hearing on legislative issues related to the regulation of dietary supplements, 29 July 1993.
3. National Nutritional Foods Association, *Natural Products Industry Fact Sheet*, 9 September 1998.
4. U. Wiedermann, X. J. Chen, L. Enerback, L. A. Hanson, H. Kahu, and U. I. Dahlgren, "Vitamin A Deficiency Increases Inflammatory Responses," *Scandinavian Journal of Immunology* 44, no. 6 (December 1996): 578–84.
5. Kuhlwein, H. J. Meyer, and C. O. Koehler, "Reduced Diclofenac Administration by B Vitamins: Results of a Randomized Double-Blind Study with Reduced Daily Doses of Diclofenac (75 mg. Diclofenac Versus 75 mg. Diclofenac Plus B Vitamins) in Acute Lumbar Vertebral Syndromes," *Klinische Wochenschrift* 68, no. 2 (January 1990): 107–15.
6. G. Bruggemann, C. O. Koehler, and E. M. Koch, "Results of a Double Blind Study of Diclofenac + Vitamin B_1, B_6, B_{12} Versus Diclofenac in Patients with Acute Pain of the Lumbar Vertebrae. A Multicenter Study," *Klinische Wochenschrift* 68, no. 2 (January 1990): 116–20.
7. G. Vetter, G. Bruggemann, M. Lettko, G. Schwieger, H. Asbach, W. Biermann, K. Blasius, R. Brinkmann, H. Bruns, E. Dorn, "Shortening Diclofenac Therapy by B Vitamins. Results of a Randomized Double-Blind Study, Diclofenac 50 mg. Versus Diclofenac 50 mg. Plus B Vitamins, in Painful Spinal Diseases with Degenerative Changes," *Zeitschrift fur Rheumatologie* 47, no. 5 (September 1988): 351–62.
8. M. Eckert and P. Schejbal, "Therapy of Neuropathies

with a Vitamin B Combination. Symptomatic Treatment of Painful Diseases of the Peripheral Nervous Sytem with a Combination Preparation of Thiamine, Pyridoxine and Cyanocobalamin," *Fortschritte der Medizin* 110, no. 29 (October 1992): 544–48.

9. Q. G. Fu, E. Carstens, B. Stelzer, and M. Zimmerman, "B Vitamins Suppress Spinal Dorsal Horn Nociceptive Neurons in the Cat," *Neuroscience Letters* 95, nos. 1–3 (December 1988): 192–97.

10. Guyton, *Textbook of Medical Physiology*, 495.

11. M. Aprahamian, A. Dentinger, C. Stock-Damilligramse, J. C. Kouassi, and J. F. Grenier, "Effects of Supplemental Pantothenic Acid on Wound Healing: Experimental Study in Rabbits," *American Journal of Clinical Nutrition* 41, no. 3 (March 1985): 578–89.

12. R. H. Davis, K. Y. Rosenthal, L. R. Cesario, and G. R. Rouw, "Vitamin C Influence on Localized Adjuvant Arthritis," *Journal of the American Podiatric Medical Association* 80, no. 8 (August 1990): 414–18.

13. D. R. Dryburgh, "Vitamin C and Chiropractic," *Journal of Manipulative Physiological Therapy* 8, no. 2 (June 1985): 95–103.

14. F. M. Gloth and J. D. Tobin, "Vitamin D Deficiency in Older People," *Journal of the American Geriatric Society* 43, no. 7 (July 1995): 822–28.

15. Robert Berkow, *The Merck Manual*, 16th ed. (Rahway, N.J.: Merck & Co., 1992), 966.

16. S. E. Edmonds, P. G. Winyard, R. Guo, B. Kidd, P. Merry, A. Langrish-Smith, C. Hansen, S. Ramm, and D. R. Blake, "Putative Analgesic Activity of Repeated Oral Doses of Vitamin E in the Treatment of Rheumatoid Arthritis. Results of a Prospective Placebo Controlled Double Blind Trial," *Annals of Rheumatoid Disease* 56, no. 11 (November 1997): 649–55.

17. Z. Mahmud and S. M. Ali, "Role of Vitamin A and E in Spondylosis," *Bangladesh Medical Research Council Bulletin* 18, no. 1 (April 1992): 47–59.

18. R. E. Newnham, "Essentiality of Boron for Healthy

Bones and Joints," *Environmental Health Perspectives* 102, S7 (November 1994): 83–85.

19. M. Benderdour, T. Bui-Van, A. Dicko, and F. Belleville, "In Vivo and In Vitro Effects of Boron and Boronated Compounds," *Journal of Trace Elements in Medical Biology* 12, no. 1 (March 1998): 2–7.

20. *The New Encyclopeadia Britannica*, 15th ed., vol. 2 (Chicago: Encyclopeadia Britannica Inc., 1991), 733.

21. Jane Brody, *Jane Brody's Nutrition Book* (New York: Bantam Books, 1987), 184.

22. Myrtle L. Brown, ed., *Present Knowledge in Nutrition*, 6th ed. (Washington, D.C.: International Life Sciences Institute, 1990), 283.

23. R. Neubauer, "A Plant Protease for the Potentiation of and Possible Replacement of Antibiotics," *Experimental Medical Surgery* 19 (1961): 143–60.

24. T. Bodi, "Modification of Tissue Permeability by Oral Bromelain in Man," *Experimental Medical Surgical Supply* (1965): 51–56.

25. G. Renzini, "The Absorption of Tetracyclin in Presence of Bromelains During Oral Application," *Drug Research* 22 (1972): 410–12.

26. S. Tinozzi and A. Vengoni, "Effect of Bromelain on Serum and Tissue Levels of Amoxycillin," *Drugs Under Experimental and Clinical Research* 4 (1978): 39–44.

27. H. Ishikawa and Y. Oguro, *Japanese Journal of Antibiotics* 27, no. 2 (1974): 118–21.

28. Amgrist Innerfield, *Enzymes in Clinical Medicine* (New York: McGraw Hill, 1960).

29. Amgrist Innerfield and A. Schwartz, "Parenteral Administration of Trypsin: Clinical Effect of 538 Patients," *Journal of the American Medical Association* 152 (1953): 597–99.

30. F. J. Sweeney, "Treatment of Athletic Injuries with an Oral Proteolytic Enzyme," *Medical Times* 93 (1963).

31. M. G. Cirelli, "Inflammation and Edema," *Medical Times* 92 (1964): 919–22.

32. P. S. Boyne and H. Medhurst, "Oral Anti-Inflammatory

Enzyme Therapy in Injuries in Professional Footballer," *Practitioner Bd* 198 (1967): 543–46.

33. J. P. Tarayre and H. Lauressergues, "Advantages of a Combination of Proteolytic Enzymes, Flavonoids, and Ascorbic Acid in Comparison with Nonsteroidal Anti-Inflammatory Agents," *Arzneim.-Forsch. Drug Research* 27 (1977): 1144.

34. Anthony Cichoke and Leo Marty, "The Use of Proteolytic Enzymes with Soft Tissue Athletic Injuries," *American Chiropractor* (September/October 1981): 32–33.

35. Rajabather Krishnaraj, "International Phytothera-peutic Uses of Garlic Food Forms," in *Nutraceuticals: Designer Foods III Garlic, Soy, and Licorice*, ed. Paul A. Lachance (Trumbull, Conn.: Food & Nutrition Press, 1997), 71.

36. Robert I-San Lin, *Garlic & Health* (Irvine, Calif.: International Academy of Health and Fitness, 1994).

37. O. M. Kandil, T. H. Abdullah, and A. Elkadi, "Garlic and the Immune System in Humans: Its Effects on Natural Killer Cells," *Federation Proceedings* 46, no. 3 (1987): 441.

38. B. H. S. Lau, "Detoxifying, Radio-Protective and Phagocyte-Enhancing Effects of Garlic," *International Clinical Nutrition Review* 9 (1989): 27–31.

39. B. H. S. Lau et al., "Garlic Compounds Modulate Macrophage and T-Lymphocyte Functions," *Molecular Biotherapy* 3 (1991): 103–7.

40. N. Takasugi, "Effect of Garlic on Mice Exposed to Various Stresses," *Oko Yakuri* (Applied Pharmacology) 28 (1984): 991–1002.

41. K. Yokoyama, "Anti-Stress Effects of Garlic Extract Preparation Containing Vitamins (Kyo-Leopin) and Ginseng-Garlic Preparation Containing Vitamin B_1 (Leopin-five) in Mice," *Oko Yakuri* (Applied Pharmacology) 31 (1986): 977–87.

42. H. Kawashima, "Anti-Fatigue Effect of Aged Garlic Extract in Athletic Club Students," *Clinical Report* 20 (1986): 111–27.

43. *Dorland's Illustrated Medical Dictionary*, 27th ed. (Philadelphia: W. B. Saunders, 1988), 276.

44. M. A. Giamberardino, L. dRagani, R. Valente, F. DiLisa, R. Saggini, and L. Vecchiet, "Effects of Prolonged L-Carnitine Administration on Delayed Muscle Pain and CK Release After Eccentric Effort," *International Journal of Sports Medicine* 17, no. 5 (July 1996): 320–24.

45. Setnikar, R. Palumbo, S. Canali, G. Zanolo, "Pharmacokinetics of Glucosamine in Man," *Arzneimittel-Forschung* 43 (1993): 1109–13.

46. Setnikar, C. Giacchetti, and G. Zanolo, "Pharmacokinetics of Glucosamine in the Dog and in Man," *Arzneimittel-Forschung* 36, no. 4 (April 1986): 729–35.

47. Luke R. Bucci, "Glucosamine—A New Potent Nutraceutical for Connective Tissues," *American Academy of Osteopathy Journal* (summer 1992): 26–27.

48. T. Shibamoto, personal communication, 1993.

49. T. Shibamoto, Y. Hagiwara, and T. Osawa, "A Flavonoid with Strong Antioxidative Activity Isolated from Young Green Barley Leaves," presented at the Agricultural Chemical Society National Conference, Washington, D.C., 1992.

50. Y. Matsuoka, H. Seki, K. Kubota, H. Ohtake, and Y. Hagiwara, *Enshou* 3 (1983): 9.

51. Richard Lucas, *Secrets of the Chinese Herbalists* (Englewood Cliffs, N.J.: Prentice Hall, 1987).

NINE

1. G. Waddell, G. Feder, and M. Lewis, "Systematic Reviews of Bed Rest and Advice to Stay Active for Acute Low Back Pain," *Journal of General Practice* 47, no. 423 (October 1997): 647–52.

2. Eleanor Criswell, *How Yoga Works: An Introduction to Somatic Yoga* (Novato, Calif.: Freeperson Press, 1989).

3. Judith Lasater, "The Ten Most Important Stretches," *Yoga Journal* (May/June 1996): 91–98.

4. Esther Myers and Kim Echlin, "Awakening the Spine," *Yoga Journal* (May/June 1996): 66–73.

5. Bert H. Jacobson, Chen Ho-Cheng, Chris Cashel, and Larry Guerrero, "The Effect of T'ai Chi Chuan Training on Balance, Kinesthetic Sense, and Strength," *Perceptual and Motor Skills* 84 (1997): 27–33.

6. N. G. Kutner, H. Barnhart, S. L. Wolf, E. McNeely, and T. Xu, "Self-Report Benefits of Tai Chi Practice by Older Adults," *Journal of Gerontology* 52B, no. 5 (1997): 242–46.

7. Herman Kauz, *Tai Chi Handbook* (Garden City, N.Y.: Doubleday, 1974).

8. Alexandra Avery, *Aromatherapy and You: A Guide to Natural Skin Care* (Kailua, Hawaii: Blue Heron Hill Press, 1994), 11.

9. J. R. Basford and M. A. Smith, "Shoe Insoles in the Workplace," *Orthopedics* 11, no. 2 (February 1988): 285–88.

10. William H. Philpott and Sharon Taplin, *Biomagnetic Handbook: A Guide to Medical Magnets, the Energy Medicine of Tomorrow* (Choctaw, Okla.: Enviro-Tech Products, 1990).

11. Janet G. Travell and David G. Simons, *Myofascial Pain and Dysfunction* (Baltimore: Williams & Wilkins, 1983).

12. George J. Goodheart, *Applied Kinesiology Research Manuals* (Detroit: George J. Goodheart, 1964–71).

13. David S. Walther, *Applied Kinesiology, Synopsis* (Pueblo, Colo.: Systems DL Publishing Co., 1988).

14. Fred Stoner, *The Eclectic Approach to Chiropractic* (Las Vegas: F. L. S. Publishing Co., 1976).

15. Toru Namikoshi, *Shiatsu Therapy, Theory and Practice* (Tokyo: Japan Publications, 1974).

TEN

1. Robert Berkow, *The Merck Manual*, 16th ed. (Rahway, N.J.: Merck & Co., 1992), 1334.

2. Ibid., 1305.

3. C. Steffen, J. Smolen, K. Miehlke, I. Horger, and J. Menzel, "Enzyme Treatment in Comparison with

Immune Complex Determinations in Rheumatoid Arthritis," *Zeitschrift fur Rheumatologie* 44 (1985): 51–56.

4. U.S. Department of Health and Human Services, *The Surgeon General's Report on Nutrition and Health* (Washington, D.C.: U.S. Department of Health and Human Services, 1988), 313–18.

5. J. O. Brynhildsen, E. Bjors, C. Skarsgard, and M. L. Hammar, "Is Hormone Replacement Therapy a Risk Factor for Low Back Pain Among Postmenopausal Women?" *Spine* 23, no. 7 (April 1998): 809–13.

6. S. Dudeney, D. O'Farrell, D. Bouchier-Hayes, and J. Byrne, "Extraspinal Causes of Sciatica. A Case Report," *Spine* 23, no. 4 (February 1998): 494–96.

APPENDIX A

1. Anthony J. Cichoke, *Introduction to Chiropractic Health* (Los Angeles: Keats Publishing, 1996).

2. J. A. Astin, "Why Patients Use Alternative Medicine: Results of a National Study," *Journal of the American Medical Association* 279, no. 19 (May 1998): 1548–53.

3. Erin Hoover Barnett, *The Oregonian*, 24 August 1998.

4. Jim Hill, *The Oregonian*, 29 April, 1999.

Suggested Reading and Viewing

ACUPRESSURE

Duo, Gao. *Chinese Medicine*. New York: Thunder's Mouth Press, 1997.

Heinke, Dagmar-Pauline. *Relieving Pain with Acupressure*. New York: Sterling Publishing, 1998.

Hin, Kuan. *Chinese Massage and Acupressure*. New York: Bergh Publishing, 1994.

Young, Jacqueline. *Acupressure for Health*. New York: Thorsons/Harper Collins, 1994.

ALTERNATIVE HEALTH

Balch, James F., and Phyllis A. Balch. *Prescription for Nutritional Healing*. Garden City Park, N.Y.: Avery Publishing Group, 1997.

Burton Goldberg Group, eds. *Alternative Medicine: The Definitive Guide*. Puyallup, Wash.: Future Medicine Publishing, 1993.

Cichoke, Anthony J. *Introduction to Chiropractic Health*. Los Angeles: Keats Publishing, 1996.

Goldberg, Isreal, ed. *Functional Foods, Designer Foods, Pharmafoods, Nutraceuticals*. New York: Chapman & Hall, 1994.

Klatz, Ronald, and Robert Goldman. *Anti-Aging Secrets*. Chicago: Elite Sports Medicine Publications, 1996.

Murray, Michael T., and Joseph E. Pizzorno. *An Encyclopedia of Natural Medicine*. Rocklin, Calif.: Prima Publishing, 1991.

Page, Linda Rector. *Healthy Healing*. Carmel Valley, Calif.: Healthy Healing Publications, 1997.

Sinatra, Stephen T. *Heartbreak and Heart Disease*. Los Angeles: Keats Publishing, 1996.

APPLIED KINESIOLOGY

Goodheart, George J. *Applied Kinesiology Research Manuals*. Detroit: George J. Goodheart, 1964–71.

Stoner, Fred. *The Eclectic Approach to Chiropractic*. Las Vegas: F. L. S. Publishing Co., 1976.

Walther, David S. *Applied Kinesiology, Synopsis*. Pueblo, Colo.: Systems DL Publishing Co., 1988.

BACK CARE

Kramer, J. *Intervertebral Disk Diseases*. Chicago: Year Book Medical Publishers, 1981.

Goldberg, Burton, et al. *Chronic Fatigue, Fibromyalgia, & Environmental Illness*. Tiburon, Calif.: Future Medicine Publishing, 1998.

CHINESE HERBAL MEDICINE

Fratkin, Jake. *Chinese Classics*. Boulder, Colo.: Shya Publications, 1990.

———. *Chinese Herbal Patent Formulas*. Boulder, Colo.: Shya Publications, 1986.

Hart, Carol, and Magnolia Goh. *Traditional Chinese Medicine*. New York: Essential Healing Arts, 1997.

Hsu, Hong-Yen. *How to Treat Yourself with Chinese Herbs*. Los Angeles: Keats Publishing, 1993.

Lee, William. *Herbal Love Potions*. Los Angeles: Keats Publishing, 1991.

Mindell, Earl. *Earl Mindell's Herb Bible*. New York: Simon & Schuster, 1992.

Mowrey, Daniel. *The Scientific Validation of Herbal Medicine*. Los Angeles: Keats Publishing, 1991.

Ramholz, James. *Shaolin and Taoist Herbal Training Formulas*. Chicago: Silk Road Books, 1992.

Reid, Daniel. *Chinese Herbal Medicine*. Boston: Shambhala, 1987.

———. *The Tao of Health, Sex, and Longevity*. New York: Simon & Schuster, 1989.

ENZYMES

Cichoke, Anthony J. *The Complete Book of Enzyme Therapy.* Garden City Park, N.Y.: Avery Publishing Group, 1999.

————. *Bromelain: The Active Enzyme That Helps Us Make the Most of What We Eat.* Los Angeles: Keats Publishing, 1998.

————. *Enzymes: Nature's Energizers.* Los Angeles: Keats Publishing, 1997.

————. *Neurologic Considerations in Toxic, Metabolic, and Nutritional Disorders.* Portland, Oreg.: Seven Seas Publishing, 1996.

————. *New Hope for AIDS.* Portland, Oreg.: Seven Seas Publishing, 1995.

————. *Enzymes and Enzyme Therapy: How to Jump Start Your Way to Lifelong Good Health.* Los Angeles: Keats Publishing,1994.

————. *Acute Trauma and Systemic Enzyme Therapy.* Portland, Oreg.: Seven Seas Publishing, 1993.

————. *A New Look at Chronic Disorders and Systemic Enzyme Therapy.* Portland, Oreg.: Seven Seas Publishing, 1993.

————. *A New Look at Enzyme Therapy.* Portland, Oreg.: Seven Seas Publishing, 1993.

Gardner, M. L. G., and K. J. Steffens, eds. *Absorption of Orally Administered Enzymes.* Berlin: Springer-Verlag, 1995.

Glenk, Wilhelm, and Sven Neu. *Enzyme.* Munich: Wilhelm Heyne Verlag, 1990.

Howell, Edward. *Enzyme Nutrition: The Food Enzyme Concept.* Wayne, N.J.: Avery Publishing Group, 1985.

Lopez, D. A., R. M. Williams, and K. Miehlke. *Enzymes: The Fountain of Life.* Charleston, S.C.: The Neville Press, 1994.

Wolf, Max, and Karl Ransberger. *Enzyme Therapy.* Los Angeles: Regent House, 1972.

Wrba, Heinrich, and Otto Pecher. *Enzyme-Wirkstoffe der Zukunft Mit Der Enzym-Therapie das Immunsystem.* Zurich: Orac, 1993.

FASTING, DETOXIFICATION, AND EXCRETION

Anderson, Richard. *Cleanse and Purify Thyself*. Tucson: Arise and Shine, 1988.

Bragg, Paul. *The Miracle of Fasting*. Santa Barbara, Calif.: Health Science, 1985.

Ehret, Arnold. *Rational Fasting*. Simi, Calif.: Lust Enterprises, 1971.

Gray, Robert. *The Colon Health Book*. Reno: Emerald Publishing, 1986.

Jensen, Bernard. *Tissue Cleansing Through Bowel Management*. Escondido, Calif.: Jensen Enterprises, 1981.

Page, Linda Rector. *Detoxification*. Carmel Valley, Calif.: Healthy Healing Publications, 1997.

Shelton, Herbert. *Fasting Can Save Your Life*. Chicago: Natural Hygiene Press, 1964.

Walker, N. W. *Colon Health: The Key to a Vibrant Life*. Phoenix: O'Sullivan Woodside & Co., 1979.

HERBS

Duke, James. *CRC Handbook of Medical Herbs*. Boca Raton, Fla.: CRC Press, 1985.

Lucas, Richard. *Secrets of the Chinese Herbalists*. Englewood Cliffs, N.J.: Prentice Hall, 1987.

Lust, John. *The Herb Book*. New York: Bantam Books, 1974.

Mindell, Earl. *Earl Mindell's Herb Bible*. New York: Fireside Books, 1992.

JUICING

Calbom, Cherie, and Maureen Keane. *Juicing for Life*. Garden City Park, N.Y.: Avery Publishing Group, 1992.

Heinerman, John. *Heinerman's Encyclopedia of Healing Juices*. West Nyack, N.Y.: Parker Publishing, 1994.

Lee, William H. *The Book of Raw Fruit and Vegetable Juices and Drinks*. Los Angeles: Keats Publishing, 1982.

Null, Gary, and Shelly Null. *The Joy of Juicing*. New York: Golden Health Publishing, 1992.

MAGNETIC THERAPY

Becker, Robert O., and Gary Selden. *The Body Electric, Electromagnetism and the Foundation of Life*. New York: Morrow, 1985.

Washnis, George J., and Richard Z. Hricak. *Discovery of Magnetic Health*. Rockville, Md.: The NOVA Publishing Co., 1993.

MASSAGE (SEE ALSO SHIATSU)

Young, Jacqueline. *Self-Massage: The Complete 15-Minutes-a-Day Massage System for Health and Self-Awareness*. New York: Thorsons/Harper Collins, 1992.

POSITIVE MENTAL ATTITUDE

Hay, Louise. *Heal Your Body: The Mental Causes for Physical Illness and the Metaphysical Way to Overcome Them*. Carson, Calif: Hay House, 1994.

Peale, Norman Vincent. *The Power of Positive Thinking*. New York: Ballantine Books, 1996.

———. *Stress Without Distress*. Philadelphia: Lippincott, 1974.

Selye, Hans. *Inspiration*. New York: Pocket Books, 1955.

REFLEXOLOGY

Dougans, Inge, with Suzanne Ellis. *The Art of Reflexology*. New York: Barnes & Noble Books, 1995.

Superzem, Wolfgang. *Foot Reflexology*. New York: Sterling Publishing, 1998.

SHIATSU

Endo, Ryokyu. *Tao Shiatsu, Life Medicine for the Twenty-First Century*. Tokyo: Japan Publications, 1995.

Namikoshi, Toru. *Shiatsu Therapy, Theory, and Practice*. Tokyo: Japan Publications, 1974.

Serizawa, Katsusuke. *Massage, The Oriental Method*. Tokyo: Japan Publications, 1972.

TAE-BO

Basic Tae-Bo. Hollywood: Tae-Bo. [7095 Hollywood Blvd., Hollywood, CA 90028, 1-800-637-8820] Videotape.

Instructional Tae Bo. Hollywood: Tae-Bo. [7095 Hollywood Blvd., Hollywood, CA 90028, 1-800-637-8820] Videotape.

Advanced Tae Bo. Hollywood: Tae-Bo. [7095 Hollywood Blvd., Hollywood, CA 90028, 1-800-637-8820] Videotape.

8-Minute Workout. Tae-Bo [7095 Hollywood Blvd., Hollywood, CA 90028, 1-800-637-8820] Videotape.

TAI CHI

Kauz, Herman. *Tai Chi Handbook.* Garden City, N.Y.: Dolphins Books, Doubleday, 1974.

Kuo, Simone. *Long Life, Good Health Through Tai Chi Chuan.* Berkeley, Calif.: North Atlantic Books, 1991.

Lau, Paul. *Tai Chi.* New York: The Video Collection, Wellsprings Media, 1995. [65 Bleecker Street, New York, NY 10012] Videotape.

Ross, David-Dorian. *T'ai Chi Ch'uan.* Portland, Oreg.: New Age Fitness, 1995. Videotape.

Sun, Wei Yu, and William Chen. *Tai Chi Ch'uan.* New York: Sterling Publishing, 1995.

TRADITIONAL CHINESE MEDICINE OR TAOISM

Beinfield, Harriet, and Efrem Korngold. *Between Heaven and Earth.* New York: Ballantine Books, 1991.

Blofeld, John. *Toaism: The Road to Immortality.* Boulder, Colo.: Shambhala, 1978.

———. *Taoist Mystery and Magic.* Boulder, Colo.: Shambhala, 1982.

Chuen, Lam Kam. *The Way of Energy: A Gaia Original.* New York: Fireside/Simon & Schuster, 1991.

Cleary, Thomas. *Awakening to the Tao.* Boston: Shambhala, 1988.

———. *I Ching: The Book of Change.* Boston: Shambhala, 1992.

————. *The Inner Teachings of Taoism*. Boston: Shambhala, 1988.

————. *Vitality, Energy, Spirit*. Boston: Shambhala, 1992.

Deng, Ming-Dao. *The Wandering Taoist*. San Francisco: Harper & Row, 1983.

Kaptchuck, Ted J. *The Web That Has No Weaver*. New York: Congdon & Weed, 1983.

Lin, Yutang. *The Wisdom of China*. New York: Modern Library, 1963.

Needham, Joseph. *Science and Civilization in China*. Vol. 2. Cambridge: Cambridge University Press, 1954.

Porter, Bill. *Road to Heaven*. San Francisco: Mercury House, 1993.

Reid, Daniel P. *The Tao of Health, Sex, and Longevity*. New York: Simon & Schuster, 1989.

Waley, Arthur. *The Way and Its Power: A Study of the Tao The Ching and Its Place in Chinese Thought*. New York: Grove Press, 1958.

Welch, Homes. *Taoism: The Parting of the Way*. Boston: Beacon Press, 1957.

Wilhelm, Richard, and Cary Baynes. *The I Ching or Book of Changes*. Princeton, N.J.: Princeton University Press, 1966.

Wong, Eva. *Cultivating Stillness*. Boston: Shambhala, 1992.

WEIGHT LOSS

Simontacchi, Carol. *Your Fat Is Not Your Fault*. New York: Penguin Putnam, 1997.

YOGA

Criswell, Eleanor. *How Yoga Works (An Introduction to Somatic Yoga)*. Novato, Calif.: Freeperson Press, 1989.

Living Arts. Books, videotapes, clothes, and accessories. P.O. Box 2939, Venice, CA 90291 or can be ordered by calling 1-800-254-8464.

Reid, Daniel. *The Complete Book of Chinese Health and Healing*. Boston: Shambhala, 1995.

Yoga Journal. Yoga books, videotapes, clothes, and accessories. 1-800-2-LIVING.

A

B

U

ulcers	57
ultrasound	223
urea	91
urinary retention	58

V

valerian	143
Vander Kolk, Charles	85
vertebrae	
defined	10, 11, 12
fractures of	30–31
vertebral curves	11
Vigorous Vegetable	
Powerhouse	97
Vishnudevananda	185
visualization	
(conceptualization)	
about	80
exercises for	
back pain	80, 81–82
techniques for	83
vitamin A	111
vitamin B complex	111–13
vitamin C	113
vitamin D	113–14
vitamin deficiencies	
about	60–61, 62
and back pain	49, 49–50
vitamin E	114–15
vitamin K	115
vitamins	103, 110–15

W

water, importance of	98
water balance changes	59
Watts, Alan	78
weight lifting	180
Western diet	109
Western medicine	16, 19
whiplash	28, 30
white willow	143–44
wild cherry	144
wild yam	144
wintergreen	144
Wobenzym, N.	128
wrinkling	53

Y

yarrow	144
yin and yang	22
yoga	
cobra	187–88
corpse	186–87
fish	187
half locust	188
level of difficulty	160
yoga, tai chi and	
qi gong, about	78
Yoga Journal	
"Awakening the	
Spine,"	189
"Ten Most Important	
Stretches,"	189

Z

zinc	119